The British Medical Association

FAMILY DOCTOR GUIDE *to*

FOOD & NUTRITION

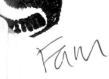

The British Medical Association

FAMILY DOCTOR GUIDE *to*

FOOD &
NUTRITION

Dr. Joan Webster-Gandy

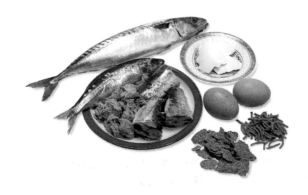

MEDICAL EDITOR
Dr. Tony Smith

A DORLING KINDERSLEY BOOK

IMPORTANT

This book is intended not as a substitute for personal medical advice but as a supplement to that advice for the patient who wishes to understand more about his/her condition.

Before taking any form of treatment YOU SHOULD ALWAYS CONSULT YOUR MEDICAL PRACTITIONER.

In particular (without limit) you should note that advances in medical science occur rapidly and some of the information about drugs and treatment contained in this book may very soon be out of date.

PLEASE NOTE
The author regrets that she cannot enter into any correspondence with readers.

DORLING KINDERSLEY
LONDON, NEW YORK, SYDNEY, DELHI, PARIS,
MUNICH AND JOHANNESBURG

DK www.dk.com

Senior Editor Mary Lindsay
Senior Art Editor Janice English
Production Controller Heather Hughes

Managing Editor Martyn Page
Managing Art Editor Bryn Walls

Produced for Dorling Kindersley Limited by
Design Revolution, Queens Park Villa,
30 West Drive, Brighton, East Sussex BN2 2GE
Editorial Director Ian Whitelaw
Art Director Becky Willis
Editor Julie Whitaker
Designer Fiona Roberts

Published in Great Britain in 2000 by
Dorling Kindersley Limited,
9 Henrietta Street, London WC2E 8PS

2 4 6 8 10 9 7 5 3 1

A CIP catalogue record for this book is available from the British Library

ISBN 07513 0621 5

Reproduced by Colourscan, Singapore
Printed in Hong Kong by Wing King Tong

Contents

Introduction

The food you eat has a strong influence on your health and on your chances of developing disease and some types of cancer. This book is aimed at people who are basically healthy, to help them understand nutrition and choose a diet that will keep them in good health.

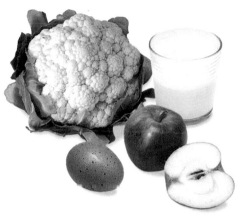

This book starts with detailed information about how you digest food. The following five chapters explain your need for energy, protein, fat, carbohydrates and vitamins and minerals, and look at their functions within your body. These chapters include the science of nutrition, good food sources and links with illnesses, such as heart and bowel diseases and cancer.

A chapter on 'Healthy eating' (see p.63) enables you to put the information together so that you can plan a diet that incorporates appropriate amounts of the various food groups. It also includes information on the safest and most effective way to lose weight.

To make informed choices about your diet, you need to know how to read the nutritional labelling on food packets, and to be aware of the various ways in which fresh produce may have been treated to make it more acceptable to consumers. These topics are covered under 'Food labelling' (see p.73) and 'Food additives' (see p.80).

EATING FOR HEALTH
A nutritionally balanced diet that includes plenty of fruit and vegetables will have a beneficial effect on your health.

Some people cannot eat certain foods or food additives for health reasons, even foods that are essential to a balanced diet. Information on this aspect of nutrition is covered in 'Food allergies and intolerances' (see p.87).

There are many different nutritional products and diets available. These are claimed to enhance a balanced diet or encourage rapid weight loss, and are covered in 'Supplements, diets and "health foods"' (see p.93).

This book provides an overview of nutrition. For people requiring further information on specific medical conditions or nutritional requirements (for example, vegans), see the list of useful addresses (p.100).

KEY POINTS

- Diet has a strong influence on your health and on your chances of developing heart disease and some cancers.

- This book is designed for people who are primarily healthy, but who wish to understand nutrition and follow a diet that will keep them in good health.

How your body uses food

Everything that goes into your stomach is mixed with enzymes, chemicals that break food into its basic components. This mixture is then passed from your stomach into your intestines, where the nutrients are absorbed into your bloodstream. The nutrients are transported around your body to the cells where they are used or stored. Food components that are not absorbed are excreted.

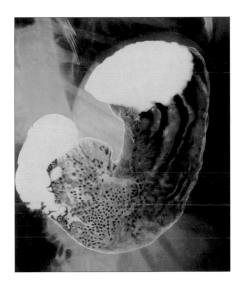

THE DIGESTIVE TRACT
The stomach is an essential element in the digestive system, storing and helping to break down the food that we eat.

— YOUR GASTROINTESTINAL TRACT —

Your gastrointestinal (digestive) tract, which runs from the mouth to the anus, is a tube of approximately seven metres in length.

YOUR MOUTH AND STOMACH

Digestion begins as soon as you start chewing food. Saliva, which is secreted by glands in your mouth, is mixed with the food as you chew it to make it easier to swallow. Saliva contains the enzyme amylase, which breaks down starchy carbohydrate foods into simpler sugars that can be absorbed into your body. Amylase can work only in an alkaline environment.

Once food is swallowed, it travels down your oesophagus (gullet) to your stomach. At its entrance and exit, your stomach has rings of muscle called sphincters, which act as valves. When food arrives at your stomach, the top sphincter opens, so that food can enter. The top sphincter then closes, keeping the food and digestive juices inside your stomach. If this sphincter leaks, digestive juices, including acid, are regurgitated into your gullet. When this happens, you experience heartburn, as your stomach's acid contents irritate the lining of your oesophagus.

Digestive juices are added to food from glands in your stomach wall. These juices contain chemicals that break down food into a usable form. Two of these chemicals are the enzyme protease (which breaks down proteins) and hydrochloric acid (which destroys most of the bacteria present in food and provides the acid conditions in which protease works). The only substance that is not subject to these digestive processes is alcohol, which is absorbed into your bloodstream directly from your stomach.

Your stomach acts as a reservoir. Semi-liquid food remains there for 2–4 hours before being released in small amounts through the bottom sphincter into your small intestine.

YOUR SMALL INTESTINE

This is the longest part of your gastrointestinal tract, being 5–6 metres long. It is called the 'small' intestine as it is narrow, only 2–4 centimetres in diameter, compared with the large intestine, which is six centimetres in diameter. Your small intestine consists of three distinct parts. Your duodenum lies just after your stomach, and is the shortest

The Digestive Process

Food must be broken down for the body to absorb and use its nutrients. As food passes through the body, it is broken down into its basic components by enzymes. Undigested waste is excreted via the anus.

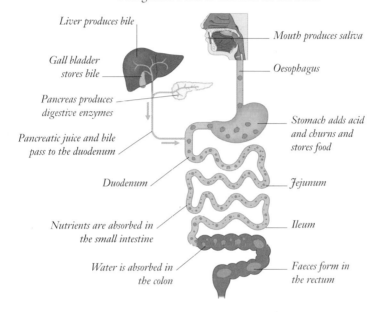

Liver produces bile

Mouth produces saliva

Gall bladder stores bile

Oesophagus

Pancreas produces digestive enzymes

Stomach adds acid and churns and stores food

Pancreatic juice and bile pass to the duodenum

Duodenum

Jejunum

Nutrients are absorbed in the small intestine

Ileum

Water is absorbed in the colon

Faeces form in the rectum

part of your small intestine. It is followed by your jejunum and your ileum, which connects to your large intestine.

When food enters your duodenum, it is still acid from the stomach juices. Alkaline digestive juices are now added to neutralise it. These are produced in an organ lying below your stomach called the pancreas and contain enzymes that continue to digest food. Bile is also added to the mixture. This green, watery fluid, which is produced in your liver and stored in your gallbladder, helps to keep fatty material in solution.

Villi of the Small Intestine

The intestinal wall is covered with millions of tiny projections, called villi. These villi provide a surface though which nutrients can be absorbed.

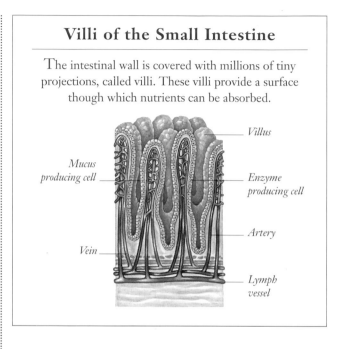

Villus

Mucus producing cell

Enzyme producing cell

Artery

Vein

Lymph vessel

Once the digestive juices have done their job, the main food components are broken down into their constituents:

- Proteins into amino acids.
- Carbohydrates into glucose and other simple sugars.
- Fat into fatty acids and glycerol.

Further down your small intestine, in your jejunum and ileum, the end-products of digestion are absorbed through the intestinal wall into your bloodstream. Food is passed along your intestine by wave-like contractions of muscles in your intestinal wall; this is called peristalsis. Your intestinal wall is not smooth, but consists of millions of tiny finger-like protrusions called villi. The villi give your intestines a large surface area through which food is absorbed. Water-soluble vitamins and minerals are also absorbed at this stage of digestion.

Once the nutrients have been absorbed, the remaining undigested food passes through another sphincter muscle into your large intestine. Your body can store some nutrients, such as those providing energy and certain vitamins and minerals. Excesses of nutrients that cannot be stored are lost in the faeces.

Your Large Intestine

Your large intestine consists of your colon, rectum and anus, and is up to a metre in length. It reabsorbs the water that is used in digestion and eliminates undigested food and fibre. Once water has been reabsorbed in your colon, the faeces, which are now drier and more solid, are passed along your rectum by peristalsis and are finally expelled through your anus.

When faeces reach your rectum, they trigger the desire to defaecate, due to reflex contractions of your rectum and the relaxation of your anal sphincter muscles. Your anal sphincters are circular muscles that control the opening and closing of your anus.

It usually takes 1–3 days for food to pass from your mouth to your anus. Some people defaecate 2–3 times a day, others daily and some only every 2–3 days. All of these patterns are normal.

THE IMPORTANCE OF FIBRE

Fibre, or non-starch polysaccharides (NSPs), are derived from plant material. Fibre cannot be broken down by digestive enzymes, so it passes through your gastrointestinal tract without being absorbed. As it adds bulk to your diet, fibre makes you feel full and also regulates your bowel movements. It does this by retaining water in your gut, increasing the bulk of the gut contents.

If you eat a high-fibre diet with plenty of fluids, your faeces will be bulky. As a result, they stimulate your gut wall, increasing peristalsis, and pass through more quickly and easily. This prevents constipation, which affects 10–12 per cent of the population. This figure rises to 20–30 per cent of those aged over 60. Changing to a high-fibre diet and drinking more fluids can ease constipation in most people. Laxatives should be used only on medical advice, as they are not always necessary, and their abuse can lead to other problems, such as loss of muscle tone in the bowel.

A high-fibre diet also helps prevent a common disorder called diverticular disease. The early stages of this can be detected in at least 15 per cent of people over 50. Most sufferers have a history of constipation, which leads to increased pressure in the colon. Straining to pass hard faeces can stretch the wall of the large intestine, encouraging the formation of small pouches, called diverticula, which are pushed outwards from the bowel wall. Inflammation and bacterial overgrowth in these pouches may cause pain and diarrhoea. A high-fibre diet with plenty of fluids can relieve the symptoms in most people, but some people require treatment with laxatives.

BOWEL CANCER

Fibre in the diet is also important in connection with bowel cancer, the third most common type of cancer. If detected early enough, it has a very good prognosis, but many people delay seeking medical advice due to embarrassment. A diet that is low in fibre increases the risk of developing bowel cancer. This is because, without fibre, unabsorbed food takes longer to pass through the gut. This means that the bowel lining is exposed to potentially harmful compounds in the unabsorbed food for longer periods.

Case History: **DIVERTICULAR DISEASE**

Tom, a widower in his 70s, had suffered from intermittent diarrhoea and severe pains in his lower abdomen for a couple of weeks. When his doctor questioned him about his bowel habits, it became clear that Tom suffered from constipation. Faeceal analysis showed that Tom did not have an infection. A barium enema, which gives a picture of the lining of the large intestine, showed that Tom was suffering from diverticular disease. He was referred to a dietitian. The dietitian discovered that Tom's diet did not include much fibre and that he drank only small amounts of fluid. She advised Tom on how to increase the amount of fibre in his diet, while still enjoying his favourite foods. She also encouraged him to increase his fluid intake. By following this advice, Tom was able to relieve his symptoms.

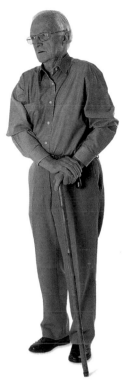

ABDOMINAL PAIN
Tom was found to be suffering from diverticular disease. By increasing his intake of fibre and liquid, he was able to alleviate his symptoms.

KEY POINTS

- Food is broken down into its building blocks by enzymes in your stomach and your small intestine.

- Nutrients are absorbed into your bloodstream from your intestine.

- Some nutrients can be stored in your body, but others are excreted.

- Fibre is essential for the normal movement of food along your bowel and has an important role in food digestion and absorption.

Energy

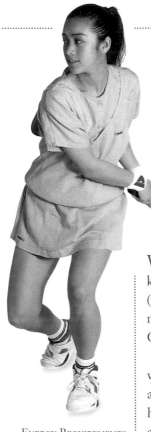

Your body's primary need, apart from water, is for energy. When your body needs energy, you feel hungry. The amount of energy you need and use is measured in calories. A thousand calories make up a kilocalorie (kcal), or Calorie (with a capital C).

When people use the word 'calorie', they mean kilocalories. Therefore, when this book refers to calories (with a small c), it refers to kcal. Energy may also be measured in joules or thousands of joules (kilojoules or kJ). One kcal is equivalent to 4.2 kJ.

Calories are often used as a negative term, with people worrying about taking in too many. When people talk about having 'lots of energy', they mean that they feel healthy. In nutritional terms, however, energy and calories are actually the same thing.

ENERGY REQUIREMENTS
People who take part in strenuous physical activities such as tennis will need more calories than those with leisurely hobbies.

WHY DO YOU NEED ENERGY?

Your body needs energy for life, voluntary activities (such as movement) and special purposes such as pregnancy, breast-feeding and growth. You need energy to breathe, digest and absorb food and maintain your body temperature. The rate at which you use energy is known as your metabolic rate. Your resting metabolic rate (RMR)

Activities and Energy Expenditure

All activities burn calories. However, the more strenuous the activity that you undertake, the more calories you burn and the greater your total energy requirement.

ACTIVITY	KCAL PER MINUTE	kJ PER MINUTE
Sitting	1.4	6
Walking slowly	3	13
Golf	2.5–4.9	10–20
Housework	2.5–4.9	10–20
Digging	5.0–7.4	21–30
Playing squash	7.5+	32+
Aerobic exercise	7–9	29–38

is the number of kilocalories or kilojoules that you use just by existing (breathing, pumping blood around your body, etc), and represents about 70 per cent of your total energy expenditure. Any activity, no matter how small (even sitting up), will use energy. The more activity you do, the more calories you burn up.

═══ HOW MUCH DO YOU NEED? ═══

The estimated average requirements (EARs) for energy show the amount of energy needed by men and women of average weights, with sedentary occupations, who do not do much exercise.

If your level of activity increases, either at work or because you start to take more exercise, your total energy requirement will increase too.

Energy Requirements for Males

The amount of daily energy that a man needs varies according to age and lifestyle. Average requirements are listed below, although there is much variation within each group.

AGE	KCAL PER DAY	MJ PER DAY
0–3 months	545	2.28
4–6 months	690	2.89
7–9 months	825	3.44
10–12 months	920	3.85
1–3 years	1,230	5.15
4–6 years	1,715	7.16
7–10 years	1,970	8.24
11–14 years	2,220	9.27
15–18 years	2,755	11.51
19–50 years	2,550	10.60
51–59 years	2,550	10.60
60–64 years	2,380	9.93
65–74 years	2,330	9.71
75+ years	2,100	8.77

Your energy requirements change at different stages of your life, for example, growth requires a lot of energy. A child will use up less energy than an adult. However, if you compare energy requirements per kilogram of body weight, a child actually uses up a higher proportion of energy per body weight than an adult.

After maturity, the adult energy requirement is fairly constant, but shows a slight, and continuing, decline after reaching the age of 30.

Energy Requirements for Females

The amount of energy that a woman needs for daily life is generally lower than that of a man. However, extra calories are needed during pregnancy and breast-feeding.

AGE	KCAL PER DAY	MJ PER DAY
0–3 months	515	2.16
4–6 months	645	2.69
7–9 months	765	3.20
10–12 months	865	3.61
1–3 years	1,165	4.86
4–6 years	1,545	6.46
7–10 years	1,740	7.28
11–14 years	1,845	7.92
15–18 years	2,110	8.83
19–50 years	1,940	8.10
51–59 years	1,900	8.00
60–64 years	1,900	7.99
65–74 years	1,900	7.96
75+ years	1,810	7.61
ADDITIONAL REQUIREMENTS	**KCAL PER DAY**	**MJ PER DAY**
PREGNANCY (THIRD TRIMESTER)	+200	+.80
LACTATION	+450–480	+1.90–2.00

Energy requirements during pregnancy increase to meet the needs of the uterus, placenta and fetus. A pregnant woman's blood volume increases and she lays down extra fatty tissue. The increase in estimated energy requirement for pregnancy in the last trimester, from around week 26,

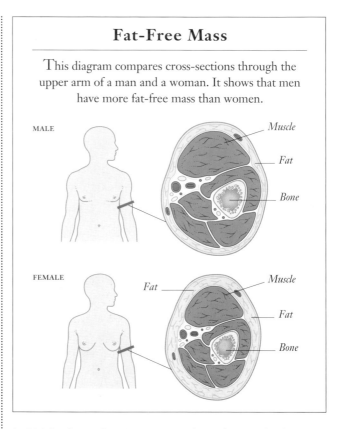

Fat-Free Mass

This diagram compares cross-sections through the upper arm of a man and a woman. It shows that men have more fat-free mass than women.

MALE

Muscle

Fat

Bone

FEMALE

Fat

Muscle

Fat

Bone

is 200 kcal per day. A woman who is breast-feeding her baby needs, on average, an extra 500 kcal per day to maintain a good supply of breast milk.

Your body weight is determined by two components: fat and fat-free mass (FFM). Fat-free mass consists of your body's lean tissues, including muscle, bone, blood and internal organs. These structures are responsible for most of your energy consumption.

The amount of FFM you have determines how many calories you use, as fat itself burns very few calories. Men have a higher proportion of FFM than women and will therefore burn more calories. This means that a man will need more calories per day than a woman of the same age and weight.

ENERGY BALANCE

If you eat the same amount of calories as you use up, your weight will remain constant. If you eat more calories than you need, your weight will increase. To lose weight, you need to use more calories than you take in.

Over a long period, any excess energy is stored as fat. If your energy intake exceeds your energy output by 7,000 kcal, you will gain 1 kilogram (2.2 pounds) in weight. It does not matter if you eat these extra calories in one sitting or over a period of days or weeks, the weight gain will be the same, although the rate of weight gain will differ. The additional weight will not be pure fat, but 75 per cent fat and 25 per cent FFM (fat-free mass). This is because extra lean tissue (for example, cell walls, blood vessels and connective tissue) is needed to support the extra fat. Most of the energy is used by FFM. Therefore, as you increase the amount of FFM in your body as you gain weight, you will use more energy.

If you continue to eat more than you need, you will continue to gain weight. To lose weight, you must eat fewer calories. As you lose weight, you lose FFM and lower your energy requirements. This means that you will have to take in even less energy if you are to continue losing weight.

When you reach your target weight, you can consume the amount of calories that will balance your energy intake with your energy expenditure and you will then stabilise at your new weight. For more on weight loss, refer to 'Healthy eating' (see pp.63–72).

Foods that Contain Approximately 100 kcal

The energy value of a food depends on the relative proportions of carbohydrate, fat, protein, alcohol and water that it contains. The following foods all contain approximately 100 kcal.

 290ml (one mug) skimmed milk

 95g potato baked in jacket

 150ml (half a mug) whole milk

 1kg cauliflower

 290 ml (approx. half a pint) lager

 50g bag of crisps

 2 slices wholemeal bread

 1½ apples

 25g Cheddar cheese

 60g chicken

 20g chocolate

 1 large egg

Energy Values

The following table gives the energy or calorific values (in kilocalories and kilojoules) of carbohydrate, fat, protein, alcohol and water – the basic food components.

NUTRIENT	KCAL PER GRAM	kJ PER GRAM
Carbohydrate	4	17
Fat	9	38
Protein	4	17
Alcohol	7	29
Water	0	0

WHERE DO YOU GET ENERGY?

Energy in your diet is provided by carbohydrate, fat, protein and alcohol. Almost all the weight of a food is made up of these components, plus water. Foods that contain a lot of water, which has no calorific value, such as many fruits and vegetables, will have less protein, fat or carbohydrate for a given weight and will therefore also be low in calories. A fatty food, such as butter, which contains relatively little water, will be rich in calories. The energy or calorific value of the food components is given in the table above.

ALCOHOL

Alcohol is a source of energy but contains no other nutrients. It is rapidly absorbed from your stomach and slowly broken down (metabolised) by your liver. The rate at which this occurs determines how quickly you become intoxicated. The rate of metabolism varies from one person to another and depends on their size. Generally,

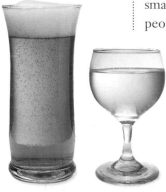

ALCOHOLIC DRINKS
Although alochol is high in energy, it contains little else of nutritional value. Intake should be restricted to the recommended number of units.

smaller people metabolise alcohol more slowly than large people, and women more slowly than men. Drinking alcohol with food will slow down the rate at which the alcohol is absorbed from your stomach, meaning that it will have a less intoxicating effect.

The maximum recommended intake of alcohol is three units a day for men and two units a day for women. A unit is about eight grams of alcohol and is equivalent to one small glass of wine, half a pint of beer or one pub measure of spirits. Drinking more than the recommended amount increases the social and physical hazards.

Recent studies have shown a relationship between moderate intakes of alcohol and a decrease in the rate of coronary heart disease. The mechanism for this is unclear, although it is thought that alcohol probably has a beneficial effect on certain types of fat in the bloodstream, which helps to stop the arteries becoming clogged.

KEY POINTS

- Your body needs energy to survive.
- Children have higher energy requirements than adults in relation to their body weight, whereas those of older people are lower.
- Fat is your body's main energy store and is used when you do not eat enough food.
- People put on weight when their energy intake exceeds their energy requirements.

Protein

Proteins are the building blocks of your body. Without them, you would not be able to replace or repair your body cells. An average 70-kilogram man contains about 11 kilograms of protein. Nearly half of this is found in skeletal muscle.

— WHY YOU NEED PROTEIN —

Protein has many important uses in your body. It is a major component of structural tissues such as skin and collagen, which are found in connective tissue such as tendons and ligaments. Blood requires protein for red blood cells, white blood cells and numerous compounds in plasma. Your body's immunity is also dependent on protein, which is needed for the formation of antibodies and white blood cells that fight disease. Enzymes and some hormones (for example, insulin) are also proteins.

If your diet does not provide enough energy, your body will eventually use functional body proteins (proteins that are incorporated into the essential structure of your body). Your body can adapt to a lack of protein in the short term. However, conditions such as injury, infection, cancer, uncontrolled diabetes and starvation can cause substantial protein losses. In these cases, the body starts to lose muscle to generate enough energy. If left unchecked, this can become life threatening.

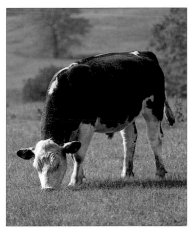

SOURCES OF PROTEIN
Meat is a major source of protein. Protein provides essential materials for body growth and repair.

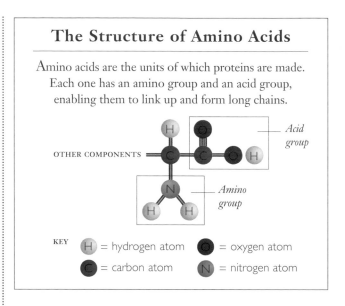

The Structure of Amino Acids

Amino acids are the units of which proteins are made.
Each one has an amino group and an acid group,
enabling them to link up and form long chains.

OTHER COMPONENTS

Acid group

Amino group

KEY H = hydrogen atom   O = oxygen atom

C = carbon atom   N = nitrogen atom

WHAT ARE PROTEINS?

Proteins are large compounds of smaller units called amino acids. Amino acids contain carbon, hydrogen, oxygen, nitrogen and occasionally sulphur. All amino acids have an acid group and an amino group attached to a carbon atom. 'Amino' is the chemical name for the combination of nitrogen and hydrogen in these compounds.

The amino group of one amino acid can link with the acid group of another amino acid to form a dipeptide. The link is called a peptide bond. When more than two amino acids join together, a polypeptide is formed. A typical protein may contain 500 or more amino acids joined together. The size and shape of each polypeptide determine what protein it is and its function. Some proteins are made of several polypeptides. Each species has its own characteristic proteins. The proteins of human muscle, for instance, are different from those of beef muscle.

How You Use Proteins

Proteins are broken down into amino acids and small peptides by enzymes (proteases) in your gut. The small peptides and amino acids are taken via your bloodstream to your liver, where they are used or transported to your body's cells. Your liver is the most important site of amino acid and protein metabolism. Amino acids are chemically changed so that they can be used for energy, converted into urea (the form in which they are excreted) or converted into other amino acids or proteins. Some proteins, such as collagen in connective tissue or tendons, are very resistant to digestion and pass through your gut unchanged to be excreted.

All the proteins your body needs can be made from 20 different amino acids. You can make some of these

Bonds Between Amino Acids

The link between two amino acids is called a peptide bond, and a chain containing more than one of these is called a polypeptide. Some proteins consist of several polypeptides and contain other kinds of bond in addition to peptide bonds.

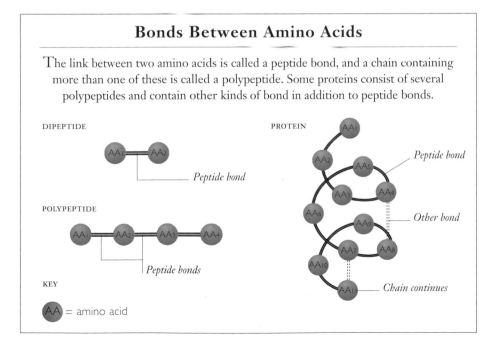

DIPEPTIDE

AA1 ——— AA2

Peptide bond

POLYPEPTIDE

AA1 ═══ AA2 ——— AA3 ══ AA4

Peptide bonds

KEY

AA = amino acid

PROTEIN

Peptide bond

Other bond

Chain continues

Sources of Protein

Meat, fish and dairy products are a good source of protein. Plant sources include cereals, beans and pasta. The foods in the table below each contain six grams of protein.

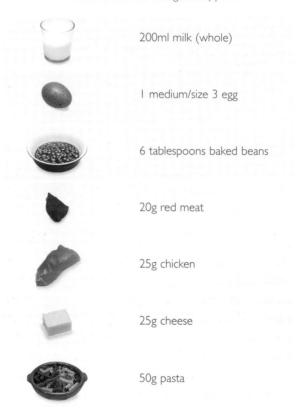

200ml milk (whole)

1 medium/size 3 egg

6 tablespoons baked beans

20g red meat

25g chicken

25g cheese

50g pasta

from other amino acids, but there are eight amino acids that cannot be made by your body and these amino acids must be supplied by your diet. These are called essential amino acids. Children need a further two amino acids for growth.

Protein Requirements

The recommended amount of protein in your daily diet is determined primarily by your age and sex. The figures set out in the table below are the estimated average requirements (EARs).

CHILDREN		MALES		FEMALES	
AGE	G PER DAY	AGE	G PER DAY	AGE	G PER DAY
< 1 year	11.0	11–14 years	33.8	11–14 years	33.1
1–3 year	11.7	15–18 years	46.1	15–18 years	37.1
4–6 years	14.8	19–50 years	44.4	19–50 years	36.0
7–10 years	22.8	50+ years	42.6	50+ years	37.2

The World Health Organization (WHO) does not give figures for 0–3 months, so no EAR can be derived. To save confusion, all babies under 1 year have been put together.

WHERE IS PROTEIN FOUND?

Protein can be found in animal produce such as meat, fish, eggs, milk and milk products, and in plant foods such as cereals, beans and pulses. All protein sources contain some of the essential amino acids, but in varying amounts. Some foods, e.g. milk and eggs, contain almost the ideal mixture of amino acids, but usually miss out one essential amino acid or contain it in inadequate amounts. It is important to eat a mixture of protein sources to ensure that you have an adequate supply of all the essential amino acids.

HOW MUCH DO YOU NEED?

The staple foods that make up the average diet in the UK have a fairly high ratio of protein to energy. It is very unlikely that a person whose diet provides enough energy will be deficient in protein. However, this may happen if

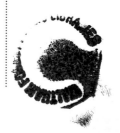

their diet contains a lot of 'empty calories', such as sugar or alcohol, which provide energy but very little protein.

SPECIAL NEEDS

There are some people, such as children, vegetarians and vegans and pregnant or breast-feeding women, who need to ensure that they have enough protein in their diet.

CHILDREN

Children need extra protein so that they can grow properly. The estimated average requirement (EAR) of a four- to six-month-old baby is more than twice that of an adult at 1.4 grams per kilogram of body weight per day. It is estimated that more than 40 per cent of an infant's protein intake should be essential amino acids. This falls to 32 per cent in pre-school children and 22 per cent in 10–12 year olds. Adults need 11 per cent.

The two extra essential amino acids that children need are found in the same protein sources as the other essential amino acids. Vegan or macrobiotic diets, which contain no animal produce including dairy products, are not suitable for small children. They are unlikely to provide all the essential amino acids. As they contain large amounts of bulky fibrous foods, these diets are unlikely to supply sufficient energy as fat or carbohydrate and, therefore, protein may be used to make up the deficit.

VEGETARIANS AND VEGANS

Provided that you follow guidelines on what constitutes a balanced diet, you can get all the essential amino acids and other nutrients you need without eating meat or fish. However, you should mix your sources of protein. Dietary guidelines vary depending on what types of food you choose to avoid. An ova-lacto-vegetarian eats animal proteins such as eggs, milk and milk products, especially cheese. A vegan who consumes only vegetable sources of protein may find it harder to ensure that they get all the necessary nutrients, but it certainly isn't impossible. It is advisable to make sure you know how to balance your diet properly before becoming a vegan. There are various books available and the Vegan Society produces information and product lists.

If you are bringing your child up as a vegetarian, it is important to make sure that your child's energy needs are met. Weaning foods such as pulses, cereals, bananas and avocado pears should be given frequently. The timing of the introduction of some foods should follow current guidelines, for example, wheat should not be introduced before one year of age. Aim to include two different plant sources of protein at each meal because this will provide a better balance of amino acids. It will probably be necessary to supplement your child's diet with vitamins and minerals. This should ideally be done in consultation with health professionals, such as a health visitor or dietitian.

PREGNANT AND BREAST-FEEDING WOMEN

A pregnant woman needs an extra six grams of pure protein daily to allow her baby to develop properly. This will also meet her own needs, which increase as she develops extra body tissues. Breast-feeding is very demanding in terms of both energy and protein. To maintain an adequate milk supply, which is a rich source of protein, it is estimated that the mother requires an extra 11 grams of protein per day from birth until her baby is six months old, and eight grams extra per day afterwards.

If you are on a strict vegan or macrobiotic diet, you may need iron and vitamin supplements while pregnant or breast-feeding. Babies should not routinely be given soya milk because it is not supplemented with the necessary vitamins and minerals. You should discuss your diet and that of your baby with a dietitian.

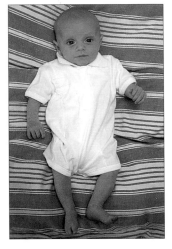

FAILURE TO THRIVE
Breast-fed babies need a good supply of breast milk to thrive. Sue's milk lacked certain essential nutrients, probably as a result of her macrobiotic diet.

Case History: **ANAEMIA**

Polly was born at full term and weighed 2.5kg (5lb 8oz). Her mother Sue follows a macrobiotic diet and would like to bring up Polly to eat the same way. Sue breast-fed Polly and introduced solids when she reached five months. Polly began to sleep poorly, and her weight did not increase appreciably from the time she started on solids. Sue's health visitor arranged a referral to the paediatrician at the local hospital. Investigations showed that Polly was anaemic and deficient in iron and vitamin B12. It is likely that, as a result of her diet, Sue's breast milk was lacking in both these nutrients. The paediatric dietitian advised Sue on how to wean Polly and maintain adequate nutrition on a vegetarian diet. She emphasised that strict macrobiotic diets are not suitable for children under two years old.

KEY POINTS

- Proteins are made of amino acids.
- Essential amino acids cannot be made in your body and, therefore, need to be obtained from food.
- Vegetarian diets can be suitable for all age groups, but vegan diets are not suitable for children, especially those under school age.

Fats

Fats (or lipids) in your diet are often divided into two types: visible and invisible. Visible fats are those that are obvious, such as butter, margarine, cooking oils and fat on meat. Invisible (hidden) fats are incorporated during cooking (for example, in cakes and biscuits) or during food preparation (as in sausages). Emulsions of fat are used extensively in products such as mayonnaise. Some foods, such as eggs, are also rich in fat.

WHY DO YOU NEED FAT?

A lot is written about the harmful effects of fat. However, fat is an essential part of your diet for three reasons.

• **Palatability** Fat makes many foods taste better. It is no use a food being nutritious if people do not like it and therefore will not eat it.

• **Energy** Fats are a concentrated source of energy, providing nine kcal per gram (38 kJ per gram).

• **Essential nutrients** Fat in your diet provides fat-soluble vitamins (for more details, see 'Vitamins and minerals' on p.52) and essential fatty acids.

VISIBLE FATS
Fats can be grouped into 'visible fats', such as olive oil and butter, and 'invisible fats', which are incorporated during cooking and food manufacturing.

WHAT ARE FATS?

The basic building blocks of fat are fatty acids and glycerol. A fatty acid is made up of a chain of carbon atoms with an acid group at one end and a methyl group at the other. A methyl group consists of one carbon atom and two hydrogens. Three different fatty acids combine with glycerol to form a triglyceride. The fat in your food is made up of a mixture of triglycerides.

Saturated and Unsaturated Fatty Acids

If each carbon atom in the chain that makes up a fatty acid is attached to two hydrogen atoms, the fatty acid is said to be saturated. If hydrogen atoms are missing, it is said to be unsaturated.

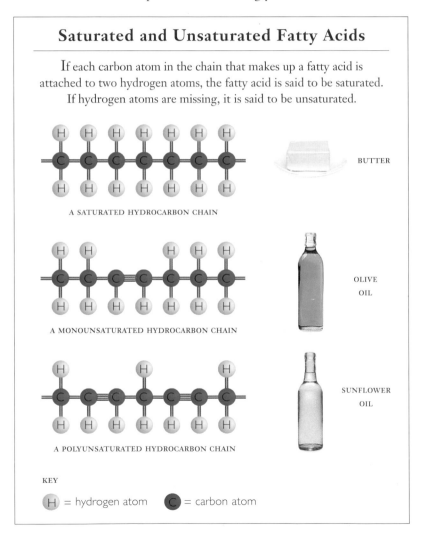

A SATURATED HYDROCARBON CHAIN

BUTTER

A MONOUNSATURATED HYDROCARBON CHAIN

OLIVE OIL

A POLYUNSATURATED HYDROCARBON CHAIN

SUNFLOWER OIL

KEY

H = hydrogen atom   C = carbon atom

The amount and type of fatty acids you eat influences the way in which your body handles them and therefore their role in diseases such as coronary heart disease. Each carbon atom in a fatty acid chain is attached to one or two hydrogen atoms. If the fatty acid has all the hydrogen atoms that it can hold, it is said to be saturated.

If, however, some hydrogen atoms are missing, the fatty acid is said to be unsaturated. In unsaturated fats, the missing hydrogen atoms are replaced by a double bond between the carbon atoms.

All fats contain both saturated and unsaturated fatty acids, but their relative proportions give fat its predominant characteristics (for example, oil or solid). The level of saturation of a fat is also referred to as hydrogenation. It is possible to alter this level of saturation (or hydrogenation) in the manufacture of fats and oils.

SATURATED FATS

Generally, fats that originate from animal sources, such as butter, have a high level of saturation. Saturated fats are more solid at room temperature than unsaturated fats.

UNSATURATED FATS

Unsaturated fats are derived from vegetable sources. Monounsaturated fats have two hydrogen atoms missing from the fatty acid complex and therefore have one double bond.

Polyunsaturated fatty acids have more than two hydrogen atoms missing and, therefore, have more than one double bond.

The less saturated the molecule, the more liquid it will be. There are exceptions to this, such as coconut oil, which is a saturated fat but is liquid. Food manufacturers have developed ways of producing unsaturated solid fats by using stabilisers and emulsifiers. When margarine was first developed in France in 1869, it was made of animal fats and was therefore a saturated fat, but today it is made from vegetable oils and chemically hardened.

ESSENTIAL FATTY ACIDS

Most fatty acids can be made in your body. However, linoleic acid and linolenic acid must be supplied by your diet. These are known as essential fatty acids (EFAs). Some others can be produced to a limited extent from these two essential fatty acids.

Essential fatty acids (EFAs) keep cell walls in good condition and working properly. They are also important in the transport, breakdown and excretion of cholesterol. They are used to manufacture other chemicals in your body such as prostaglandins. Dietary EFAs may also be involved in the brain development of babies. Most vegetable oils and oily fish are good sources of EFAs.

FATS KNOWN AS 'TRANS' FATS

'Trans' fats are produced industrially by modifying the structure of a fatty acid so that it is a mirror image of its natural form. The trans fatty acids can be found in some margarines and spreads. There is some inconclusive evidence linking these fatty acids with an increased risk of atherosclerosis and some cancers, so manufacturers are now producing margarines and spreads containing smaller amounts of trans fatty acids.

—— HOW DO YOU USE FATS? ——

Fats are insoluble in water. Therefore, they have to be emulsified by bile salts to make them accessible to digestive enzymes. This occurs to a limited extent in your stomach, but is completed in your small intestine. The presence of undigested fat in your stomach delays the rate of emptying, giving fat a 'high satiety value' and making you feel full.

Fat is broken down into smaller compounds such as cholesterol, fatty acids and glycerols. These compounds form small particles called micelles, which are small enough to be absorbed through your gut wall. In your intestinal wall, the micelles are reassembled into larger compounds and transported to your liver. Your liver then produces lipoproteins, such as high-density lipoprotein (HDL), very low-density lipoprotein (VLDL) and low-density lipoprotein (LDL). The amount of cholesterol in your diet influences the ratio of the production of these lipoproteins.

HOW MUCH FAT DO YOU NEED?

The Government guidelines on a balanced diet say that no more than 30 per cent of your total energy intake should come from fat. Saturated fat should not be responsible for more than 10 per cent of your total energy intake.

The recommended dietary intake of EFAs for adults is 1–2 per cent (2–5 grams per day) of the total energy intake and one per cent for children and babies. However, the average daily intake for adults is actually 8–15 grams of EFAs per day. EFA deficiency can occur in children and in patients requiring intravenous feeding, but it is rare in healthy individuals.

CHOLESTEROL

Cholesterol is used by your body to make steroid hormones and bile salts and to maintain the structure of cell membranes. However, raised blood cholesterol levels are associated with an increased risk of coronary heart disease (CHD). This is because cholesterol can be deposited in arteries, making them narrower – a condition known as atherosclerosis. One or more blood vessels can become totally blocked, preventing blood from reaching the tissues served by the vessel. If the blood supply is stopped, the tissue dies, and if the blocked vessel is one of the coronary arteries, the result is a heart attack. Your likelihood of developing atherosclerosis is linked to several factors including the amount of fat in your diet.

DIET AND CHOLESTEROL LEVELS

Although some foods are rich in cholesterol, most cholesterol (95 per cent) is made in your body. Your body makes cholesterol from saturated fat. The more saturated fat in your diet, the higher your blood cholesterol levels.

Polyunsaturated fats help to lower blood cholesterol. They trigger your liver to produce a phospholipid called HDL, which reduces your risk of heart disease. Eating more high-fibre food, especially soluble fibre, also helps to reduce your cholesterol levels. Soluble fibre binds with cholesterol in bile, preventing its reabsorption by your body and increasing its excretion.

There has been a lot of interest in the so-called 'Mediterranean diet', which is eaten by people in southern Europe and north Africa, who have a lower rate of CHD than in the UK. This diet is high in monoun-saturated fats. Studies suggest that these fats have little influence on

Heart Disease Risk Factors

Several factors have been found to influence an individual's risk of developing heart disease. Some risks are avoidable, others are not.

AVOIDABLE	UNAVOIDABLE
Diet	Genetic disposition
Smoking	Gender
Obesity	Age
Stress	
Lack of exercise	

blood cholesterol. The benefits of the 'Mediterranean diet' appear to derive from the fact that it is low in total and saturated fat and high in fruits, vegetables and wine.

Low levels of cholesterol have been linked to an increased risk of cancer. In fact, cancer rates are no higher in populations with low cholesterol levels than they are in those with high levels. Any disadvantages of a low-cholesterol diet are outweighed by its benefits in reducing the risk of coronary heart disease.

Case History: RISK OF CHD

George, aged 50, moved home because of his job. The local health centre where he registered as a new patient required him to have a health check. This showed that he had several risk factors for coronary heart disease (CHD), including: a family history of CHD, his age and gender, his stressful job and lifestyle, smoking, being overweight, raised blood pressure and raised blood lipid levels.

The dietitian at the health centre suggested ways in which George could modify his lifestyle and reduce his risk factors for CHD. The first priority was to reduce George's weight, which he did by following a low-fat, high-fibre diet of no more than 1,500 kcal a day. This diet was designed to help him maintain a healthier weight and reduce his blood lipids. The practice nurse also encouraged George to take suitable exercise and advised him on how to cut his stress levels and stop smoking.

Six months later, George had reduced his weight by two stone and as a result, his blood pressure was now normal. The changes in his diet and lifestyle resulted in a reduction in his blood

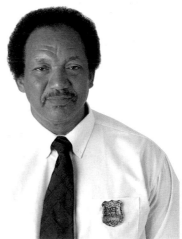

BEING OVERWEIGHT
George's excess weight contributed to his high blood pressure and greatly increased his risk of developing heart disease.

lipids. The changes George had made over the previous six months had greatly reduced his risk factors for CHD and he was feeling fitter and more energetic than he had for a long time.

KEY POINTS

- Fat is an essential part of your diet.
- Cutting down on your total fat intake, especially of saturated fat, is better than trying to substitute one kind of fat for another.
- Fat should provide a maximum of 30 per cent of your total daily calories.

Carbohydrates

Carbohydrates are your main source of energy. When they are combined with oxygen (oxidised) in cells, carbon dioxide and water are formed and energy is released.

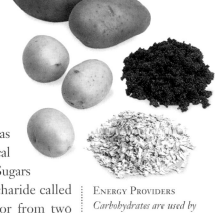

Carbohydrates are classified by nutritionists as sugars, starches and fibre. Their basic chemical structure is a compound called a saccharide. Sugars are formed either from a single type of saccharide called a monosaccharide (for example, glucose) or from two saccharides joined together forming a disaccharide (for example, sucrose). When many saccharides are joined together, polysaccharides are formed (for example, starch).

ENERGY PROVIDERS
Carbohydrates are used by the body for energy. Sugars are simple carbohydrates. Starches in potatoes and cereals need to be broken down before they can be absorbed by the body.

SUGARS

Sugars are important sources of dietary energy. Glucose is used as fuel by your body's cells, and your brain is almost entirely dependent on it for all its functions, including thinking.

Excess sugars are stored in your liver as glycogen. These stores are mobilised if you are not getting enough energy from your diet or if energy is needed quickly for exercise. If these stores are full, sugars are converted into fat and stored in adipose tissue. Your body is able to regulate the levels of glucose in your blood. If you eat a lot of carbohydrate, your pancreas produces more of the hormone insulin, which encourages the conversion of sugars into glycogen, returning your blood glucose levels to normal. When you exercise, you use more glucose and need less insulin.

WHAT ARE SUGARS?

There are two main types of sugar: monosaccharides and disaccharides. Monosaccharides are simple sugars composed of only one type of saccharide, such as glucose, fructose and galactose. Disaccharides are combinations of two monosaccharides, and include sucrose, lactose and maltose. Disaccharides are broken down by digestive enzymes in your intestine and reabsorbed as monosaccharides. For example, sucrose is broken down to glucose and fructose.

INTRINSIC SUGARS
Sugars that occur naturally in foods are known as intrinsic sugars. Good sources include honey, fruit and vegetables.

WHERE IS SUGAR FOUND?

Sugars are found in a variety of foods. Those occurring naturally in the structure of foods are called intrinsic sugars; those added in the production process are called extrinsic sugars.

Glucose is found in small amounts in fruit and vegetables, such as grapes and onions, and, with fructose, is one of the main constituents of honey. Free glucose is not a common natural sugar, but is produced commercially from starch. Fructose is found in fruit, vegetables and honey. Galactose, when combined with glucose, is found in milk. Other monosaccharides include mannose, pentose and ribose. Sucrose is the most commonly used disaccharide, and is extracted commercially from sugar beet or sugar cane. It is present in fruit and vegetables, but table sugar, which is 99 per cent pure sucrose, is the major source in the diet. Maltose consists of two glucose units and is produced commercially by breaking down starch. It is present in malted wheat and barley, which are used to produce malted foods and in the brewing industry to make beer. Lactose is found naturally only in milk and milk products. It consists of glucose and galactose.

Food manufacturers use many sugars in foods. All of the following are sugars or sugar-related products: glucose, fructose, galactose, lactose, invert sugar, mannose, pentose, ribose, sucrose, maltose, sorbitol, mannitol, dulcitol, inositol, corn syrup, trehalose, raffinose, stachyose, vernanose and fructans.

Commercial sugar comes in many forms, including white, granulated, caster, icing, demerara, cane, soft brown, dark brown, treacle, golden syrup, molasses and cubes. The stage and type of processing determines the colour and form of the sugar. None of these sugars contain substantial amounts of any other nutrients.

Sugar alcohols, such as sorbitol, are compounds that are sweet but have the same chemical structure as alcohol. Sorbitol is found naturally in some fruits, such as cherries, but it is also made commercially from glucose.

HOW MUCH SUGAR IS NEEDED?

Recent surveys show that sugars provide 18 per cent of the total energy intake for the average adult. The intake of 'refined' or 'added' sugars may contribute to the development of obesity and may limit the intake of other more beneficial foods, especially fibre. Sugars contribute energy but no other nutrients to the diet, and are therefore often called 'empty calories'. Current thinking is to reduce the amount of energy from sugar to no more than 10 per cent of dietary energy.

DENTAL DISEASE

Sugars in the diet have been linked to dental disease. Dental plaque is the white layer that builds up on teeth between brushings. Plaque is made of bacteria, water, polysaccharides and sometimes dead cells from your mouth. It collects in areas that are difficult to clean; these are often called food traps. Sugars from food pass into the plaque and are changed into acid by bacteria. The acid starts to dissolve the hard enamel coating of your teeth, causing tooth decay or dental caries. When the acid is neutralised, your tooth can heal, but a frequent intake of sugars maintains the acid environment, stopping the healing process.

Tooth Decay

Tooth decay has penetrated the hard enamel covering of the tooth and invaded the dentin, the softer material that makes up the bulk of the tooth.

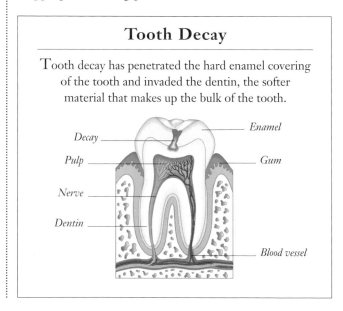

Decay

Pulp

Nerve

Dentin

Enamel

Gum

Blood vessel

People who eat large amounts of refined sugars, such as sucrose, have the most dental decay. The more frequent the intake of refined sugars, the greater the number of cavities found. There is no evidence to suggest that intrinsic sugars, such as fructose in fruit and lactose in milk and milk products, have any adverse effects on teeth. However, the use of fruit juices in comforters (dummies), which maintain prolonged periods of contact with teeth, can contribute to decay. There is strong evidence to suggest that extrinsic sugars, such as sucrose, are involved in the development of dental decay.

STARCHES

Starchy foods are an important part of your diet. In some parts of the world, starch provides up to 80 per cent of the total energy intake. In the UK, starch provides about 24 per cent of the total energy intake.

WHAT IS STARCH?

Starch is a large, complex compound (a polysaccharide) that is made up of many glucose molecules. The glucose can combine in many different ways or patterns, and this affects the rate at which you digest and absorb starch. The more complicated the pattern, the more resistant the starch will be to digestion. Raw starch is very difficult to digest. Processing, such as cooking, can change the patterns of glucose molecules, making the starch more digestible. Heating starch in water causes it to swell and thicken. This allows it to be broken down by the digestive enzyme amylase into glucose, which can be absorbed into your body.

STARCHY FOODS
Complex carbohydrates, or starches, are formed by a long chain of saccharide molecules and are found in potatoes, root vegetables and cereals.

45

Starchy Foods

Starches are complex carbohydrates. They are found in many plant foods. The following foods provide good sources of starch:

Potatoes	Rice
Bread	Biscuits
Pasta	Popcorn
Baked beans	

SOURCES OF STARCH

In the UK, the major sources of starches in the diet are staple foods such as potatoes, cereal grains (wheat, barley, maize, oats and rye) and rice. The following ingredients are also forms of starch: amylopectin, dextrins, maltodextrins and glycogen.

HOW MUCH DO YOU NEED?

Although there is no official recommendation for starches, a healthy diet should provide an average of 37 per cent of energy from starches, intrinsic sugars (which occur naturally in produce) and milk sugars. The same is true for children over two years. The best nourishment for babies is breast milk, which does not contain starch.

DIABETES

Rapidly absorbed carbohydrates, such as sucrose, result in high glucose levels in the blood. Healthy people are able to cope with this by adjusting their insulin production accordingly. Insulin is a hormone, secreted by the pancreas, that helps to move glucose from the blood into the body's cells.

If you have diabetes, this mechanism does not work. The aim of diabetic control is to maintain blood glucose levels within normal limits. People with diabetes either do not produce insulin and need to inject it (insulin-dependent diabetes mellitus or type 1 diabetes) or produce insulin but are resistant to its action (non-insulin-dependent diabetes mellitus or type 2 diabetes).

Either way, they cannot deal effectively with a rapid rise in blood glucose. High levels of glucose in the blood result in the acute symptoms of diabetes, such as thirst and increased urination and, in the long term, in complications such as eye, nerve and circulatory disorders.

Not all carbohydrates are potentially harmful to people who suffer from diabetes. For example, starches are important to people with diabetes because they do not cause rapid changes in blood glucose levels, yet provide energy and fibre.

Sorbitol is often used in products manufactured for people with diabetes. It is 60 per cent as sweet as sucrose, is absorbed slowly from the gut and is then stored as fructose in the liver. It has less effect on blood glucose levels than sucrose. However, sorbitol has more calories per gram and too much of it can give you diarrhoea. People with diabetes do not actually need a sucrose substitute and they could do without the extra calories it provides as well. The British Diabetic Association does not recommend the use of special diabetic food products to its members.

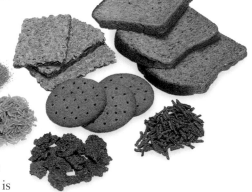

INSOLUBLE FIBRE FOODS
Wholemeal bread, biscuits, and cereals are examples of insoluble fibre foods. Insoluble fibre is not broken down in the intestine.

FIBRE

Fibre was originally called roughage and is now referred to as non-starch polysaccharides (NSPs).

Technically, dietary fibre is difficult to define and analysing foods for their fibre content can be problematic. Government bodies have recommended that the term 'non-starch polysaccharides' be used in food labelling. However, as fibre is the term that most people are familiar with, it is used throughout this book.

WHAT IS FIBRE?

Fibre is the major component of plant cell walls and is resistant to enzymes that digest food. Most of the fibre in the diet come from fruit, vegetables and cereals. In wheat, maize and rice, the fibre is mainly insoluble, whereas in oats, barley and rye, it is mainly soluble. In fruit and vegetables, the ratio of insoluble to soluble fibre is variable. Each kind of fibre plays a different role in digestion.

Insoluble fibre increases the bulk and wetness of faeces. It therefore prevents and relieves constipation by holding water in your bowel. The increased bulk speeds up the transit time of faeces and reduces the pressure in your bowel. The reduction in pressure helps prevent a condition called diverticular disease (for more details, see 'How your body uses food' p.9).

SOLUBLE-FIBRE FOODS
Good sources of soluble fibre include oats, baked beans, lentils, peas and many fruits.

Soluble fibre has little effect on stool bulk. However, it binds bile acids, which are rich in cholesterol. The cholesterol found in bile is usually reabsorbed into your body. Soluble fibre prevents this reabsorption so more cholesterol is lost in the faeces and less is take back into your bloodstream. This can be important in the prevention of coronary heart disease.

The digestion and absorption of carbohydrates are slower if there is a good supply of fibre in your diet. This results in a more gradual release of glucose into your blood, which is especially important for people with diabetes. Fibre makes you feel full because once it has absorbed water it has a larger bulk.

Soluble and Insoluble Fibre

Insoluble fibre passes through the intestine unchanged whereas soluble fibre is partly broken down by bacteria in the intestine. The following foods are examples of each type:

SOLUBLE FIBRE	INSOLUBLE FIBRE
Beans, for example, baked beans	Wholemeal bread
	Wholemeal breakfast cereals
Lentils	
Peas	Wholemeal biscuits and crisp breads
Oats	
	Brown rice
Oranges	Wheat bran
Apples	Oats

HOW MUCH FIBRE DO YOU NEED?

A recent Government panel recommended that the adult diet should contain 12–24 grams of fibre per day from a variety of sources. This amount could be provided by five portions of fruit and vegetables per day.

There is no specific recommendation for children besides suggesting that fibre intake should be related to body size, so children need proportionately less than adults. Children under the age of two should not be given fibre at the expense of energy-rich foods that are needed for growth.

Generally, foods rich in fibre have more bulk, are less energy dense and are more likely to reduce hunger than fibre-free foods. This suggests that they can play a useful role in weight-reducing diets.

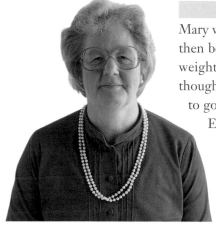

MANAGING DIABETES
By following a healthy eating plan, Mary managed to lose weight and maintain normal glucose levels.

Case History: **DIABETES MELLITUS**

Mary was a keen tennis player until she retired. She then became more sedentary and gradually put on weight. She noticed that she was always tired and thought that it was, at least partly, because she had to go to the toilet at least twice during the night, Eventually, Mary consulted her GP, who asked her for a urine sample. Using a simple dipstick test, the doctor found that Mary had a lot of glucose in her urine. He then did a finger-prick test, which showed that her blood glucose level was also high.

Mary was diagnosed with non-insulin-dependent diabetes mellitus (type 2 diabetes). This could be treated by a change of diet, with or without tablets. A dietitian analysed Mary's normal diet and felt that Mary was eating too much refined sugar and fat. She suggested a healthy eating plan. Mary needed to control her energy intake so as to lose weight. She needed to eat a variety of foods and have regular meals and snacks. She needed to eat less fat, eat more fruit and vegetables – ideally five portions a day – and include more fibre in her diet.

The dietitian also told Mary that there was no need to use products made especially for people with diabetes. These contain ingredients that are low in glucose but high in other refined carbohydrates or contain sweeteners such as sorbitol.

Once Mary's weight returned to normal, her diabetes improved greatly. She was able to monitor her glucose levels by using simple blood and urine tests. When Mary was feeling less tired, she joined the local tennis club. Regular exercise improved her general health and made it easier for her to control her blood glucose levels.

KEY POINTS

- Carbohydrate is an important source of energy in your diet.

- Try to eat more carbohydrate foods and reduce the fat content of your diet.

- Complex carbohydrates (starches and fibre) make you feel full.

Vitamins and minerals

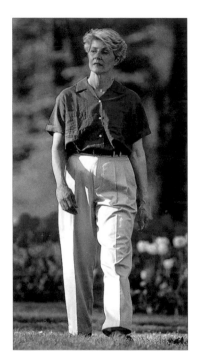

Vitamins and minerals are an essential part of a balanced diet. They are needed by your body in minute amounts for many vital chemical reactions, such as extracting energy from food. They are often called micronutrients. A lack of vitamins or minerals can lead to ill-health and cause deficiency diseases.

SUNLIGHT AND VITAMIN D
Walking in the sunlight will boost the body's natural supply of vitamin D. The sun's ultraviolet rays act on the skin to produce vitamin D.

VITAMINS

Vitamins were originally known by letters of the alphabet, but now researchers and other health professionals more often use their chemical names. Since the end of the last century, the understanding of vitamins and their role in human health and deficiency syndromes has increased greatly. Recent research has shown that they may also play a part in preventing diseases such as cancer.

WHAT ARE VITAMINS?

Vitamins are complex chemical substances. Most cannot be made in your body, so you have to obtain them from food. One exception is vitamin D, which can be made in your skin on exposure to sunlight. Bacteria, which live inside your gut, can also make some vitamins.

Vitamins can be split into two groups: water-soluble and fat-soluble. Water-soluble vitamins can be dissolved in water and, therefore, are found in non-fatty water-rich foods such as fruit and vegetables. Fat-soluble vitamins are found in fatty foods, as their chemical structures allow them to be dissolved in fat.

Some vitamins, particularly water-soluble vitamins, are gradually lost from foods over time. For this reason, the fresher the foods, and the less they are cooked, the better the supplies of vitamins available. Vitamin C, for example, is destroyed by heat, and vitamin B_1 (thiamine) is sensitive to light.

Frozen vegetables are often better sources of vitamins because they are frozen very soon after harvest and the vitamins are preserved. Fresh vegetables may be in transit or in the shop for days before being sold and may be stored at home before the food is used.

How Much Do You Need?

Only small amounts of each vitamin are required each day. There are recommended daily allowances (RDAs) for several vitamins in the UK, including thiamine, folate, riboflavin, niacin, vitamins A, B_6, B_{12}, C and D. The RDA is the required level of intake needed to maintain good health. It varies between different groups of people; infants, children, elderly people, adults and pregnant and breast-feeding women all require different amounts. For more details on vitamin supplements, see 'Supplements, diets and "health foods"' on pp.93–99.

Water-soluble Vitamins

The B-complex vitamins and vitamin C are water-soluble. Any excess is usually excreted via the urine.

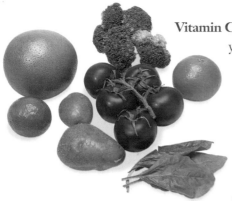

VITAMIN C FOODS
Fresh fruits and vegetables are good sources of vitamin C. Vitamin C is vital for the formation of collagen, which is important for the growth and repair of body tissues.

VITAMIN B₁ FOODS
Thiamine, is found in both animal and plant foods. Good sources include pork, nuts, peas and beans.

Vitamin C (ascorbic acid) Vitamin C helps to maintain your skin and connective tissue and helps iron to be absorbed from your gut. People who do not get enough vitamin C develop a condition called scurvy, which causes fatigue, bleeding and poor wound healing. Vitamin C deficiency is rare in healthy individuals, but can affect people with illnesses such as cancer, malabsorption syndromes and alcoholism, or those who are being fed intravenously. Vitamin C is found in fruit and vegetables, especially citrus fruit, tomatoes, spinach, potatoes and broccoli. It is easily destroyed by heat and light, so foods rich in vitamin C should be stored in a cool, dark place, and prepared and cooked as quickly as possible.

Taking high doses of vitamin C has been claimed to reduce your chances of catching the common cold. Apart from its now accepted role in preventing damage caused by free radicals, other claims have not been proved. Taking too much vitamin C can be harmful, causing diarrhoea and kidney stones. As vitamin C increases iron uptake, taking too much can also lead to iron overload.

Vitamin B₁ (thiamine) Thiamine helps to break down carbohydrate, fat and alcohol. People who have a thiamine deficiency (known as beri-beri) cannot process carbohydrates or fat properly and develop a range of symptoms including cardiac and neurological problems. In the UK, the condition mainly affects people with chronic disease, malabsorption problems or anorexia. Chronic binge-drinking alcoholics can also develop thiamine deficiency.

Most of the thiamine in the diet comes from fortified cereals and bread. Other major sources are offal, pork, nuts and legumes (peas and beans). Large doses of thiamine, in excess of three grams per day, may cause headaches, insomnia, weakness and skin problems.

Vitamin B₂ (riboflavin) Your body needs vitamin B_2 to extract energy from fat, protein and carbohydrate in food. The main sources of riboflavin are dairy products, meat, fish, asparagus, broccoli, poultry and spinach. Some cereals are fortified with riboflavin. Riboflavin is sensitive to ultraviolet light. Riboflavin deficiency can cause skin disorders, especially in and around the mouth. There is no evidence that riboflavin has toxic effects on the body, or that large doses do any good.

VITAMIN B₂ FOODS
Also known as riboflavin, vitamin B2 is found in meat, poultry, fish, asparagus, spinach, dairy products and liver.

Vitamin B₆ (pyridoxine) Pyridoxine is essential for the metabolism of proteins and haemoglobin (the oxygen-carrying red pigment in your blood), so the quantity you need depends on how much protein you eat. Pyridoxine deficiency causes skin problems in and around the mouth and neurological problems, but this rarely affects healthy people. Bacteria in your gut make pyridoxine, some of which is absorbed through your intestinal wall. Poultry, fish, pork, eggs and offal are rich sources of pyridoxine, as are oats, peanuts and soybeans.

Pyridoxine supplements are taken by many women to treat premenstrual symptoms, but there is no conclusive evidence showing that they have a beneficial effect.

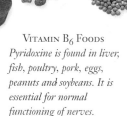

VITAMIN B₆ FOODS
Pyridoxine is found in liver, fish, poultry, pork, eggs, peanuts and soybeans. It is essential for normal functioning of nerves.

Vitamin B_{12} (cyanocobalamin) Cyanocobalamin is involved in the production of red blood cells. Foods derived from animals (including dairy products) are a good source of vitamin B_{12}. Strict vegetarians and vegans may need to take supplements to make up for any deficiency in their diets.

To be able to use vitamin B_{12}, your stomach must produce a substance called intrinsic factor. People who have a stomach disorder preventing them from making enough intrinsic factor cannot absorb vitamin B_{12} properly and they develop pernicious anaemia. There is no evidence that taking large doses of vitamin B_{12} does any harm.

Folate (folic acid) Folate is essential for the normal formation of red blood cells. People with folic acid deficiency may develop megaloblastic anaemia in which the red blood cells are enlarged. Sources of folates include liver, yeast extract and green, leafy vegetables. A good supply is important for women who are planning to conceive and those who are in the first three months of pregnancy, when the recommended intake is 400 micrograms per day. Folate has been shown to reduce the risk of having a baby with a neural tube defect such as spina bifida. High intakes of folate are not dangerous, but they may affect the absorption of zinc and interfere with tests used to diagnose vitamin B_{12} deficiency.

Unless you are planning to conceive or are in early pregnancy, there are no proven benefits from taking large doses.

FOLIC ACID FOODS
The main sources of folic acid are green leafy vegetables, yeast extract and liver. It is needed for the formation of red blood cells.

Niacin Niacin is involved in fat metabolism and is necessary to maintain the condition of your skin. Niacin deficiency is rare in developed countries, but in Asia and Africa it results in a condition called pellagra, which can be fatal if untreated. Meat is a good source of niacin and cereals provide moderate amounts. Niacin can also be made in your body from the amino acid tryptophan. Excess niacin is excreted in your urine, although very large doses can cause liver problems.

Panthothenic acid and biotin Pantothenic acid and biotin are involved in fat and carbohydrate metabolism and are found in foods derived from animal sources and in cereals and pulses. There are no recommended intakes and they are not known to be toxic.

FAT-SOLUBLE VITAMINS
Vitamins A, D, E and K are fat-soluble. Fat soluble vitamins are stored in the liver or in fatty tissue.

Vitamin A (retinol) Vitamin A can be made in your body from substances called beta-carotenes, which are found in dark-green, orange and yellow vegetables such as spinach and carrots. Retinol is obtained from animal sources, such as meat and dairy products. Deficiency is rare in the UK, but is a major cause of blindness in children in some developing countries. Retinol is toxic in large doses but most damage is done by accumulation. Toxicity can lead to liver and bone damage and cause birth defects. You should not take supplements or eat large quantities of liver just before or during pregnancy.

VITAMIN A FOODS
Beta-carotene, which is converted to vitamin A in the body, is present in yellow-orange and dark green vegetables and fruits.

57

Vitamin D (calciferol) Vitamin D is important in the growth and maintenance of bone because it controls the absorption of calcium and phosphorus, which are essential in bone metabolism. Children who do not get enough vitamin D develop rickets; adults develop weak, soft bones, a condition known as osteomalacia. Sources of vitamin D include fatty fish, such as pilchards, sardines, mackerel and tuna, eggs and fortified foods such as margarine and some breakfast cereals. Vitamin D can be made in your skin by ultraviolet rays in sunlight. Deficiency is rare in the UK, but does occur in people who have little vitamin D in their diet and whose skins are rarely exposed to sunlight – e.g., elderly people and some Asian women. Large doses can lead to high blood levels of calcium, especially in children, and may result in bone malformations, although this is extremely rare. There are no dietary recommendations for adults who have a normal lifestyle involving exposure to sunlight.

VITAMIN D FOODS
Fatty fish, eggs, margarine and breakfast cereals will boost your supply of vitamin D, which is essential for healthy bones.

Vitamin E (tocopherol) Tocopherol acts as an antioxidant, which means it stops your body's cells being attacked by chemicals called oxygen-generated free radicals. Vitamin E is important in maintaining the structure of lipids in your body and any structures, such as membranes surrounding cells, that are rich in lipids. Deficiency in humans is rare, occurring only in premature babies and in people with some malabsorption syndromes. Dietary sources include vegetable oils, nuts, vegetables and cereals. There is little evidence of tocopherol toxicity.

VITAMIN E FOODS
Vegetable oils, wholegrain cereals, vegetable and nuts are among the best sources of vitamin E.

Vitamin K (phylloquinone, menaquinone and menadione) The three forms of vitamin K have a slightly different chemical make-up. Vitamin K is involved in blood clotting and a deficiency will lead to bruising and excessive bleeding. Deficiency is rare except in newborn babies and people who have diseases affecting vitamin absorption or metabolism. Dark-green, leafy vegetables are the major sources in the diet, although bacteria in your gut can make vitamin K, which is absorbed into your blood.

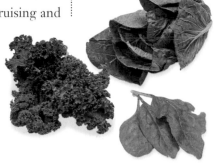

VITAMIN K FOODS
Dark-green, leafy vegetables are the best dietary source of vitamin K. Vitamin K is necessary for normal blood clotting.

MINERALS

Minerals are single chemical elements that are involved in various processes in your body. If you eat a varied diet, you should obtain all the minerals you need. Unlike vitamins, minerals do not deteriorate during storage or cooking, so mineral deficiency is rare, except in people being intravenously fed or with certain diseases. One exception is iron deficiency, which is often the result of blood loss or may develop in people who are strict vegetarians or vegans. Your body is able to adapt to make the most of its mineral supplies; for example, your iron absorption increases if your diet is poor in iron. This is why taking mineral supplements may cause problems: overloading with one mineral may decrease the absorption of another that is absorbed in your body via the same route.

OTHER MINERALS AND TRACE ELEMENTS
Sodium, potassium and chromium are also referred to, in solution, as electrolytes. They are widely distributed throughout your body and have many functions,

including maintaining your nerves in proper working order. Deficiencies and high levels of these chemicals are usually caused by a problem with a person's metabolism – for example, certain diseases or dehydration caused by excessive vomiting. Electrolytes are readily available in animal and vegetable foods.

Other minerals and trace elements used by your body include aluminium, antimony, boron, bromine, cadmium, lithium, nickel, sulphur and strontium. They are readily available in your diet and, as their name suggests, are only necessary in trace (tiny) quantities.

ANTIOXIDANTS AND DISEASE

Recently, there has been evidence that some vitamins and the mineral selenium may act as defences against certain diseases. When oxygen is used in chemical reactions in your body, it produces, as a by-product, potentially harmful chemicals called free radicals. These cause tissue damage and may lead to some conditions such as heart disease and some cancers. Your body has powerful defence mechanisms to prevent such damage, but in some cases (for example, in smokers), this mechanism is impaired. Antioxidants, such as vitamin A, beta-carotene, vitamins C and E and selenium, are able to stop the action of free radicals.

INHIBITING FREE RADICALS
Fruits and vegetables contain a good supply of antioxidants. Antioxidants can help combat the damage caused by free radicals.

Diseases linked to free radical damage occur for many reasons. However, eating a diet that is rich in antioxidant foods can reduce your risk of developing them. A recent Government committee has recommended that the best way of ensuring that you get enough of the relevant nutrients is to eat five portions of fruit and vegetables a day. Some reports have suggested that people who eat large quantities of red meat are especially at risk, although the reason for this is unclear; it may be, that people who eat a lot of meat also tend to eat fewer fruit and vegetables and are not protected against free radical damage.

Case History: OSTEOMALACIA

Henry (aged 80) lived alone and was totally house-bound. A helper shopped and cleaned for him and prepared a snack lunch each day. Henry rarely cooked a meal and found fruit difficult to eat because of his dentures. He dismissed the aches and pains in his bones and muscles as 'old age'.

One morning, Henry slipped getting out of bed. His home help found him on the floor unable to move. At the hospital, it was discovered that he had fractured the top of his thigh bone, a type of fracture that is most common in elderly people. Blood tests showed that Henry had abnormally low levels of calcium and vitamin D. A bone scan confirmed that Henry was suffering from osteomalacia. Undoubtedly, his poor diet contributed to his condition, but an important factor was his lack of exposure to sunlight, which triggers the production of vitamin D.

A dietitian gave Henry advice on which foods to eat. Social services arranged transport to a local day care centre, where he would have a nourishing meal. Going out regularly would increase Henry's exposure to sunlight, improving his bone condition.

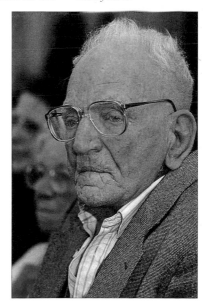

WEAK BONES
Calcium and vitamin D deficiency contributed to Henry's bone condition. A good diet and exposure to sunlight is essential for healthy bones.

KEY POINTS

- A balanced diet provides all the necessary vitamins and minerals for healthy adults.

- The benefits of large doses of vitamins (much higher than the recommended daily allowance) are not proven; large doses of fat-soluble vitamins can actually be harmful.

- Some people are at risk of a vitamin or mineral deficiency (for example, pregnant women and vegetarians), and may benefit from supplements of the correct dosage.

- Research has found links between a low vitamin and mineral intake and heart disease and some cancers; it is believed that five portions of fruit and vegetables per day can reduce the risk of developing these diseases.

- Taking folate supplements (400 micrograms per day) in pregnancy reduces the risk of having a baby with spina bifida.

Healthy eating

The key to eating a healthy diet is to have a balanced approach to food. There is no such thing as a 'good' or 'bad' food. It is important to view your diet as a whole. Only if your diet is unbalanced and contains too much of a 'less good' food will it become unhealthy. No food has to be forbidden in a healthy diet, except on medical grounds, although some are best kept as an occasional treat.

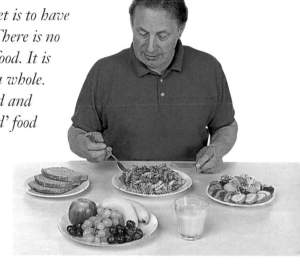

If you deny yourself a particular favourite food, you are more likely to become obsessed with it and crave it all the time. When you do succumb, you are more likely to overindulge than if you include it in your diet every now and again.

YOUR EATING PLAN

Foods should be included in your diet in the correct relative proportions. However, you do not need to measure quantities of different foods very accurately, except on medical advice. Under those circumstances, your eating pattern should be supervised by a qualified dietitian or a doctor.

There are five foods groups:
- Fruit and vegetables
- Bread, cereals, pasta and potatoes (carbohydrates)
- Meat, fish and alternatives (protein foods)
- Milk and dairy foods
- Foods containing fat or sugar.

To achieve a balanced diet, you should choose a variety of foods from the first four groups. This will supply you

Healthy Snacks

Snacks can be healthy and nutritious, as well as easy to prepare. Include foods that are low in sugar, fat and salt, and high in fibre. The easiest to prepare and most healthy snack is fresh fruit.

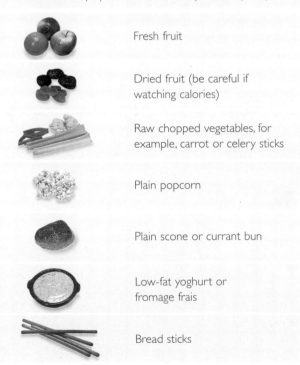

Fresh fruit

Dried fruit (be careful if watching calories)

Raw chopped vegetables, for example, carrot or celery sticks

Plain popcorn

Plain scone or currant bun

Low-fat yoghurt or fromage frais

Bread sticks

with enough of the various nutrients your body needs. Foods in the last group do not always provide a wide variety of nutrients, but can make your diet more enjoyable. They should be eaten only in moderation. Do not worry if you cannot get this balance right with every meal, but aim to do so over the course of a few days.

Aim to have three meals a day with small snacks in between if you want them. Snacks do not have to be high in calories or fat – fruit or a couple of wholemeal biscuits is a better bet. Breakfast is an important meal and should not be missed. The longer you go between meals or snacks, the more likely you are to overindulge when you next eat.

FRUIT AND VEGETABLES

Fruit and vegetables provide vitamins, minerals and fibre. The fibre can reduce constipation and help to prevent bowel disease and coronary heart disease. Fruit and vegetables are good sources of the antioxidants vitamins A and C. Recent research has shown that these substances may help prevent other diseases including some cancers. Frozen, dried and tinned fruit and vegetables are just as nutritious as fresh foods. Adults should aim to have five portions of fruit and vegetables every day; children can be given smaller portions according to their appetite.

CARBOHYDRATES

It is important to eat plenty of carbohydrates, as they are good sources of energy, fibre, calcium, iron and B vitamins. Wholemeal bread and pasta and brown rice are particularly good sources of fibre. As well as preventing constipation and bowel disease, fibre will make you feel full, helping you to stop overeating. High-fibre diets can also lower blood cholesterol, reducing the risk of coronary heart disease.

What Is a Portion?

Nutrition professionals often advise the inclusion of a certain number of portions of fruit and vegetables in the diet. This chart shows examples of the portion sizes of particular foods.

FOOD	PORTION
Apple, banana, orange	I fruit
Plums	2 fruits
Dried fruit	I tablespoon
Grapes, cherries	I cupful
Fruit juice	I small glass
Vegetables	2 tablespoons
Salad	I dessert bowlful

FAT

Fat is an essential part of your diet but you do not need very much. It provides energy, essential fatty acids and vitamins, and makes food nicer to eat. However, high levels are associated with coronary heart disease and obesity, so it is important to cut down your intake, especially when it comes to saturated fat.

You can do this by eating less 'visible' fat – such as fatty meats and eggs – and using less fat and oil for cooking and spreading. Food manufacturers offer a wide choice of low-fat products. Some products, such as cakes or biscuits, contain 'invisible' fats, so you need to read food labels carefully. Try using products that are high in polyunsaturated fats and low in saturated fats.

SUGARY FOOD AND DRINKS

These contain calories and no other nutrients, so try not to have too many of them. They are particularly harmful to your teeth and are best eaten at the end of meals.

ALCOHOL

Drinking one to two units of alcohol per day has been shown to be beneficial to health by reducing the risk of coronary heart disease. However, drinking large quantities of alcohol increases the risks to your health, and this applies even if you abstain all week and then binge at weekends.

A HEALTHY WEIGHT

You can find the appropriate weight for your height by using the chart on p.69. Your body mass index (BMI) can be calculated by dividing your weight in kilograms by your height in metres, squared.

If your BMI is less than 20, you are underweight. You should be careful not to lose any more weight and should consult your doctor. If your BMI is 20–25, your weight is in proportion to your height. If your BMI is 25–30, you are a bit overweight. Unless your health is affected (arthritis, for example, is made worse by excess weight), then you do not need to worry. If your BMI is above 30, you are overweight and should consider losing weight or your health will suffer. At BMI values greater than 30, there is an increased risk of many diseases. These include coronary heart disease (CHD), high blood pressure, some cancers, diabetes, musculoskeletal problems, reproductive disorders and gallbladder disease. If you are concerned about your weight, your GP will be able to advise you and may refer you to a dietitian or the practice nurse.

LOSING WEIGHT WISELY

To lose weight you should eat a high-fibre, low-fat diet that follows the given guidelines but has smaller portions. Once you have reached a comfortable weight that gives you a BMI below 30, you should eat a balanced diet and not have too many calories. Exercise is an important part of weight maintenance. It does not have to be strenuous but just enough to make you feel slightly out of breath – a brisk walk, for example. Aim to exercise for 20–30 minutes two or three times a week. Many GPs can now prescribe a fitness programme at the local sports centre. This may be available free or for a reduced fee.

The recommended rate of weight loss is 0.5kg (1lb) per week. If you lose weight too quickly, you may lose body tissues that are not associated with the excess weight (i.e. FFM). This will make it harder for you to maintain your new weight. You will lose more weight when you first

What Should You Weigh?

To find out whether you are a healthy weight for your height, first find your current weight on the left side of the chart below. Then run your finger across to your height and see which of the three sections you fall into.

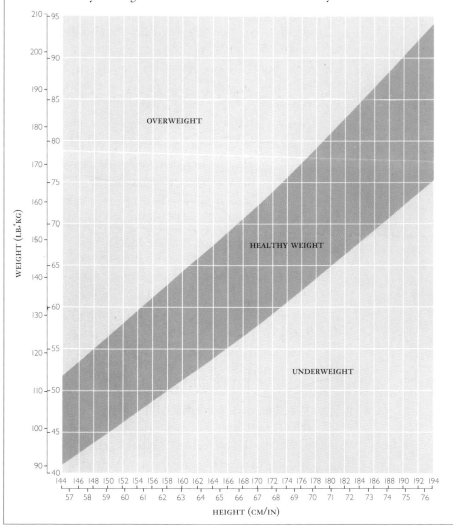

start to diet because your body uses up its stores of glycogen from your liver and muscle. Glycogen is stored with water, so as you use glycogen, you excrete a large amount of water in your urine. Glycogen is usually used up by the end of the first or second week of your diet. How much weight you lose initially will depend on the energy and carbohydrate content of your diet before you started. If you were eating a diet low in carbohydrates, your glycogen stores will be smaller than those of someone who eats large amounts.

FEEDING CHILDREN

Up to the age of four months, breast or formula milk provides all the nutrients that a baby needs. You can begin to introduce solids around this time, starting with baby rice, then puréed fruit and vegetables. Over the following weeks and months, you can gradually increase the amount and texture, so that, at 12 months, your child is eating a varied diet of three meals and two or three snacks. Introducing different textures will encourage your child to chew.

Whether you opt for bought or home-made food is a matter of personal choice. Preparing baby and toddler meals does not have to be time-consuming and fiddly, and is certainly less expensive. For example, you can make extra of a particular dish, such as fruit and vegetables, when cooking for the rest of your family. Extra portions can be puréed and frozen. Remember, however, not to add salt or sugar until your child's portion has been put into a separate dish. Keep the portions small at first. Ice cube trays make ideal containers for freezing foods. That way, not much is wasted if your baby does not like a particular food. An older toddler can be fed with the rest of your family and the food simply mashed.

Although children under two years should not eat too much fat, there is no need for them to be on a low-fat diet. They need a lot of energy to grow, some of which can be provided by fat. By the age of five, your child should be eating a balanced diet similar to that eaten by the rest of your family.

FUSSY EATERS

Some children will not eat a variety of foods or at times appear to eat very little. Although it is very frustrating for you as a parent, the best approach is to stay as calm as you can and not give your child too much attention. If you allow eating to become an issue, you will simply make the problem worse. You may be able to avoid this situation if you give your child a wide variety of foods and try to make mealtimes a relaxing and enjoyable experience.

If you are concerned about your child's diet, a referral from your GP to a paediatric dietitian may be helpful. She will be able to assess your child's diet and, with the doctor, his or her growth and development. Most fussy children are actually growing well and require little or no intervention from health professionals. Be patient and keep reminding yourself that most children grow out of this phase.

Case History: **OBESITY**

Six months after the birth of her baby, Jane started to notice that she got breathless walking upstairs and was finding coping with her baby physically more difficult. At 5 feet 4 inches (1.6 metres) and 13 stones 7 pounds (86 kilograms), she was clearly overweight, so her health visitor suggested that Jane should talk to the practice nurse. The practice nurse calculated that Jane had a BMI of 33.6, meaning she was officially classified as obese. The

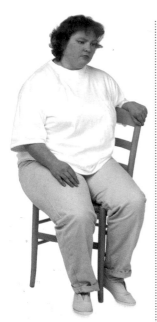

LOSING WEIGHT
Jane's increasing breathlessness and lack of energy were clearly associated with being overweight. By changing her diet, Jane gradually lost weight.

normal weight range for a woman of Jane's height is 51–64 kilograms (8–10 stone). After talking to Jane about her lifestyle and eating patterns, the nurse was able to agree on some changes with her:

- Eat three meals a day plus small snacks if necessary.
- Cut down on fatty foods, Use low-fat foods.
- Increase the amount of fibre in her diet.
- Have at least five portions of fruit and vegetables each day.
- Avoid fried food and cut down on sugar.
- Aim for a total intake of 1,400 kcal a day.

The aim was for Jane to lose approximately one pound per week after the initial period of rapid weight loss. Once her weight had dropped, Jane should try to follow the same healthy eating guidelines to ensure that she did not immediately put back what she had lost. Jane lost four pounds in the first week of her diet and was surprised that she did not feel she was depriving herself of any foods. She subsequently lost between one and one and a half pounds a week for the next month and soon felt confident to carry on without making the regular visits to the practice nurse.

KEY POINTS

- Have three meals a day and do not skip breakfast.
- There is no reason to avoid snacks.
- Eat more fibre and carbohydrate and reduce fat.
- Eat five portions of fruit and vegetables per day.
- Food should be a pleasure, not something to worry about.

Food labelling

Food labelling can help you to make informed choices about whether to include a particular food in your diet. You can now choose from a wide selection of imported fresh foods with a long shelf-life. This is partly due to improved storage methods such as refrigeration, freezing, the addition of chemicals and irradiation to delay spoiling. Before you buy food, you may wish to consider whether it has been treated to increase its acceptability and, if so, how safe these treatments are.

FOOD LABELLING LAWS

The Labelling of Food Regulations (1970) introduced requirements for claims about energy content, especially those aimed at slimmers and people with diabetes, and criteria for vitamin and mineral claims. By the mid-1980s, food manufacturers began using nutritional labelling as a marketing tool. This, and pressure from health professionals and consumers, led to further legislation. The Ministry of Agriculture, Fisheries and Food issued more guidelines in 1987 and 1991. Nutrition labelling is only mandatory when a nutrient claim is made on the label. This was in line with the directive issued by the European Union in 1993; this is due to be revised shortly.

WHAT IS IN YOUR FOOD?
By reading the labels on packaged foods, you will be able to make an informed choice about the foods you buy.

Preserving Foods

Food-preserving techniques prevent the contamination and deterioration of food. They act by inhibiting bacterial activity and the action of self-digesting enzymes that break down cells.

METHOD	HOW IT WORKS
Refrigeration	Reducing the storage temperature to 3–5°C will reduce the deterioration of fats (rancidity) and slow down microbial growth.
Freezing	Reducing the storage temperature to (18–20°C) will stop the growth of microbes, but will not kill them. Microbes will still be present, and will resume growth once the food is defrosted. It will slow the deterioration of fats even further than refrigeration, but will not stop if defrosted. This is why food should not be refrozen after thawing.
Chemicals	Alter the chemical composition of the food to reduce the impact of microbe contamination and oxidation.
Irradiation	At high doses, treating food with radiation will sterilise the food. At low doses, radiation can be used to delay ripening of fruit.

WHAT IS ON A LABEL?

As well as the name of the food, all labels should list ingredients, date by which the food should be eaten, additives, with E numbers, and nutritional information.

NAME

All pre-packed, and many non-pre-packed, foods must show the name of the food on the label. Some foods have trade names, such as Frosted Flakes, whereas others have a descriptive name, such as gravy browning. Names such as wholemeal are defined by law.

The name must be precise enough to distinguish it from other products. There are exceptions, including whole, unpeeled fresh fruit and vegetables, flavourings, cheese and butter. Names must not be misleading, for example, cherry cheesecake must have its flavour coming mainly from real cherries, as must a product with fresh cherries pictured on the packet. Cherry flavour, on the other hand, means that the product's flavour is derived mainly from artificial flavourings.

INGREDIENTS

Most foods must have the ingredients listed in descending order of weight. Water is not always included because it is often considered an integral part of food, unless it falls within the constraints of legislation. If added water takes

---

The Information on a Label

By law, food labels must provide the consumer with specific kinds of information. These include the product name, the ingredients (listed in descending order of weight) and details of the nutritional values.

CRISPBREAD

Ingredients

Wheat flour, vegetable oil, dried vegetable (sugar beet), salt

Nutritional information

TYPICAL VALUES	PER SLICE (approx 10g)	PER 100G
Energy kJ	162	1626
or Energy kcal	38	383
Protein g	1.0	9.8
Carbohydrate g	8.0	79.3
of which sugars, g	0.2	1.9
Fat g	0.4	3.8
of which saturates, g	0.04	0.4
Fibre g	0.2	2.1
Sodium g	0.04	0.4

Nutritional Claims

Some of the terms used by manufacturers to describe their products are defined in law, to avoid the possibility that consumers may be misled, but others remain vague and undefined.

FAT	Low or reduced fat	25 per cent less fat than normal product
	Fat free	Not more than 0.15g of fat per 100g
	Virtually fat free	No legal definition
ENERGY*	Reduced calorie	25 per cent less calories than normal product
	Low calorie	Not more than 40 kcal per gram or millilitre
	Diet, light or Lite	No legal definitions
SUGAR**	Sugar free	Not more than 0.2g per 100g
	Reduced sugar	25 per cent less sugar than normal product
SALT (SODIUM)	Reduced salt or sodium	25 per cent less salt than normal product
	Low salt	Not more than 40mg per serving (or 40mg per 100g serving)
	Salt free	Less than 5mg per 100g
FIBRE	High fibre	There is no legal definition of high fibre but many manufacturers use a level of at least 6g per 100g of food to mean high fibre

*Manufacturers use the phrase 'as part of a low calorie diet' to imply that a product could be useful in a slimming diet. Any food can be fitted into such a diet if intake of other food and drink is restricted. Some products are misleadingly labelled 'slimming' in that, weight for weight, they have the same or even more calories than equivalent non-slimming foods, but because they are less dense (e.g. some breakfast cereals) or are prepared in a particular way (e.g., taken in water rather than milk), the energy per serving is lower.

**No added sugar also means no honey, fructose or fruit syrup.

up five per cent or more of the finished product, it must be listed with the other ingredients. There has been a recent trend towards listing water as aqua, presumably to make it sound less ordinary.

ADDITIVES AND E NUMBERS

Ingredients that fall into this category are usually added in small quantities and therefore appear towards the end of the list. The approved name or E number may be used. An E number indicates that the additive is permitted under European Community legislation. Additives are used for flavouring, sweetening or colouring, to enhance the preservation of food or to affect its consistency or texture. Additives are discussed separately on p.80.

DATE MARK

Foods that have a shelf-life greater than three months must show a month and year by which they must be eaten. Foods with a shelf-life of less than three months must show the day and month by which they should be used. Products with a 'sell by' date rather than a 'best before' date should tell you within how many days the food should be eaten from this date. Retailers can be prosecuted for displaying products for sale after these dates.

NUTRITIONAL CLAIMS

According to voluntary guidelines issued by the Ministry of Agriculture, Food and Fisheries, nutritional values should be expressed per 100 grams of food and per portion if the packet contains less than 100 grams. It is now a legal requirement for food weights to be in grams and kilograms, although some manufacturers will quote both metric and imperial weight systems.

Information should be given about energy, protein, fat and carbohydrate, then about dietary fibre and sodium, and then about sugars, vitamins and minerals. Vitamin and mineral values are given when they are present in amounts greater than one-sixth of the recommended dietary intake.

Manufacturers who falsify claims can be prosecuted. However, the terminology used can be very confusing. For example, 'low fat' has a legal definition, but 'lower in fat' can mean anything less than normal for that product category.

▬ RECOMMENDED DAILY ALLOWANCE ▬

Nutrition labelling often includes the recommended daily allowance of energy, protein, vitamins or minerals. This is the amount that will supply the requirements of most people. There is no RDA for carbohydrate or fat because they are interchangeable sources of energy. A substance can only be listed in this way when more than one-sixth of the RDA is present.

The Government panel on the content of nutrients in the diet (Panel on Dietary Reference Values of the Committee on Medical Aspects of Food Policy, 1991) introduced two other terms: estimated average requirement (EAR) and reference nutrient intake (RNI). EAR is defined for energy, protein and vitamins for a specified group of people, for example, a specific age range. About half of this group will need more than the EAR and the other half will need less.

RNI, which is defined for protein, vitamins and minerals, is the amount that is enough for about 97 per cent of the population. For example, the EAR of women aged 19 to 50 years for riboflavin is 0.9 milligrams per day. The RNI is 1.1 milligrams per day. Most people will not need more than the EAR. However, if the average intake of riboflavin is 1.1 milligrams per day or more, at least 97.5 per cent of the population will receive enough.

These data are included on food labels for information and as a marketing tool. In everyday life, such precise knowledge is not necessary. If you are eating a balanced diet following the guidelines in 'Healthy eating' on p.63, you are unlikely to be deficient in any nutrient.

KEY POINTS

- Food labelling helps you to decide whether to buy food products, now that there is more storage, preserving and processing.

- Laws determine what nutritional claims manufacturers may make.

- The list of ingredients tells you what ingredients the food contains and in what proportions.

- RDA is the recommended daily allowance that will supply the requirements of almost everyone

Food additives

Without additives, the variety of foods available and their shelf-lives would be greatly reduced. However, the use of additives in food is a controversial subject, with claims that they can trigger allergies or are toxic. Some people are sensitive to certain additives, especially colourings, and should check food labels carefully to see what additives the food contains.

COLOURFUL ADDITIVES
Colourings are added to a variety of foods, including fizzy drinks and sweets, to make them appear more attractive to the consumer.

About 3,500 additives are in use today. The Ministry of Agriculture, Fisheries and Food is responsible for the control of additives and has a full list of them.

All permitted additives are considered safe and necessary, and are controlled by law. Food additives must gain approval before their use in food manufacture is permitted. Many additives are natural substances; for example, ascorbic acid (vitamin C) is used as a flour improver to speed up bread production. Natural additives must also undergo testing and approval before they can be used in food manufacture.

E NUMBERS

E numbers are given to permitted food additives regarded as safe for use within the European Community. Some additives have a number but no E prefix, as they are under consideration for licensing by the EC. All food labels must show the additive's name or E number in the list of ingredients.

COLOURINGS (E100–180)

Food is coloured to restore losses that occur in manufacture and storage, to meet consumer expectations and to maintain uniformity of products. An example of this is that oranges have green patches when picked and are coloured orange before sale.

PRESERVATIVES (E200–290)

Preservatives stop food going off and enable the consumer to buy a wide range of goods that are available out of the usual season. Food spoils easily: bacteria cause the structure to rot and putrify; enzymes cause unacceptable changes such as browning; injury causes some fruit cells to die, leading to discolouring and eventually rotting; fats become rancid as a result of oxidation.

Traditional preservatives include salt, vinegar, alcohol and spices. Acetic acid is the major component of vinegar and may be considered as a natural additive, but it has undergone extensive testing and has an E number (E260). Radiation can be used as a preservative because it destroys bacteria and enzymes that spoil food. It can also be used to delay ripening of fruit and sprouting in vegetables such as potatoes.

Why Use Additives?

Many of the foods we eat today contain additives. Additives are used in food for many reasons, including the following:

- To keep foods fresh until eaten, widening food choice.
- To enable food to be conveniently packaged, stored, prepared and used.
- To make the product look that much more appealing.
- To extend the food's shelf-life.
- To reduce the ingredient cost.
- To add additional nutrients.

Natural and Synthetic Colourings

Many colours are used for cosmetic reasons. About half are natural pigments, such as carbon and riboflavin. Artificial colourings such as tartrazine and amaranth are also used.

NAME	COLOUR	E NUMBER	TYPICAL USE
NATURAL COLOURS			
Riboflavin	Yellow	E101	Processed cheese
Chlorophyll	Green	E140	Fats, oils, canned vegetables
Carbon	Black	E153	Jams, jellies
Alpha-carotene	Yellow/orange	E160	Margarine, cakes
SYNTHETIC COLOURS			
Tartrazine	Yellow	E102	Soft drinks
Sunset	Yellow	E110	Orange drinks
Amaranth	Red	E123	Blackcurrant products
Erythrosine	Red	E127	Glacé cherries
Indigo carmine	Blue	E132	Savoury food mixes
Green S	Green	E142	Tinned peas, mint jelly, sauce

The radiation process is only used under licence and is monitored by a Government committee.

Other preservatives include:

● **Benzoic acid and benzoates,** which are found in many fresh foods such as peas, bananas and berries; benzoates cause adverse reactions in some people.

● **Sulphur dioxide** destroys thiamine and is therefore not permitted in foods that are a significant source of this vitamin. It is used to destroy yeasts, which can cause fermentation in food products.

Commonly Used Preservatives

*Preservatives stop or prevent the growth of microorganisms that can cause food poisoning.
The most common preservatives added to processed foods include nitrates and sulphites.*

NAME	E NUMBER	FOOD USE
Sorbic acid*	E200–E203	Cheese, yoghurt, soft drinks
Acetic acid	E260	Pickles, sauces
Lactic acid	E270	Margarine, confectionery, sauces
Propionic acid*	E280–E283	Bread, cakes, flour, confectionery
Benzoic acid*	E210–E219	Soft drinks, pickles, fruit products
Sulphur dioxide	E220	Soft drinks, fruit products, beer, cider, wine
Nitrites	E249, E250	Cured meats, cooked meats and meat products
Nitrates	E251, E252	Bacon, ham, cheese (not Cheddar or Cheshire)

*Includes derivative products.

● **Nitrates and nitrites** kill bacteria that cause botulism, a potentially lethal form of food poisoning, and preserve the red colour in meat. Nitrites may react with other chemicals in the gut to form nitrosamines, which have been shown to cause cancer in experimental animals, although there is no evidence that they do the same in people.

ANTIOXIDANTS (E300–322)
Fats and oils become rancid through oxidation, which causes an unpleasant taste and smell. The higher the fat content of a product, the faster the food becomes rancid. This process can be delayed, but not stopped, by low

83

Permitted Antioxidants

Antioxidants prevent or delay oils and fats in food from turning rancid. Some antioxidants are natural substances, such as vitamins C and E. Others are synthetic, such as BHA and BHT.

NAME	E NUMBER	FOOD USE
Ascorbic acid (vitamin C)*	E300–E305	Beer, soft drinks, powdered milk, fruit, meat products
Tocopherols (vitamin E)*	E306–E309	Vegetable oils
Gallates	E310–E320	Vegetable oils and fats, margarine
BHA	E320	Margarine and fat in baked products, e.g. pies
BHT	E321	Crisps, margarine, vegetable oils and fats, convenience foods

*Includes derivative products.

temperatures (for example, refrigeration). The use of antioxidants prevents oxidation. The most common antioxidants are butylated hydroxyanisole (BHA) and butylated hydroxytoluene (BHT).

EMULSIFIERS AND STABILISERS (E400–495)

These additives are used to increase the shelf-life of foods and affect their texture and consistency.

Emulsifiers are fatty compounds that change the chemical properties of some foods so that they can be mixed. An example of this is vinaigrette, which will normally separate out with oil floating on the top of the vinegar. If an emulsifier, such as lecithin, is added to the vinaigrette, the oil and vinegar will stay mixed together in an emulsion.

Emulsifiers and Stabilisers

Emulsifiers are used to prevent the oil and water components of many foods from separating. Stabilisers are added to improve texture, and are often made from plant matter such as seaweed.

NAME	E NUMBER	FOOD USE	CATEGORY
Lecithins*	E322	Chocolate, margarine, potato snacks	Emulsifier
Citric acid**	E472a–c	Pickles, dairy and baked products	Stabiliser
Tartaric acid**	E472d–f	Baking powder	Stabiliser
Alginic acid**	E400–E401	Ice cream, instant desserts and puddings	Stabiliser
Agar	E406	Tinned ham, ice cream	Stabiliser
Carrageenan	E407	Ice cream	Stabiliser
Gums	E410–E415	Ice cream, soups, confectionery	Stabiliser
Pectin	E440	Preserves, jellies	Stabiliser

*May also be used as an antioxidant.

**Includes derivative products.

Stabilisers (e.g. pectin) are usually large carbohydrates. They form a structure that is capable of holding the smaller chemicals in foods together, forming a more stable product. This is the largest group of additives and many are natural substances – e.g. carrageenan, which is derived from seaweed and is used as a gelling agent. Thickeners are carbohydrates that alter or control the consistency of a product during cooling or heating, or in storage. Raising agents are used to give a light spongy texture to cakes and other baked products, and include bicarbonate of soda, tartaric acid and baking powder (a mixture of sodium bicarbonate and sodium pyrophosphoric acid).

SWEETENERS

These are divided into two groups. Caloric sweeteners add energy to the diet, and include mannitol, sorbitol, xylitol and hydrogenated glucose syrup. Non-caloric sweeteners are synthetic sweeteners, and include acesulfame K, aspartame, saccharin and thaumatin. Sucrose, glucose, fructose and lactose are all classified as foods rather than sweeteners or additives.

OTHER ADDITIVES

Glazing agents are used to give food an appealing shiny appearance, and include egg-based products. Flour improvers are used to produce bread with a lighter texture and to slow staling.

Other additives include: flavour enhancers, such as monosodium glutamate (which intensifies the flavour of food); anti-foaming agents (which prevent frothing during processing); and propellant gases (which are used, for example, in aerosol cream). Polyphosphates enable products to retain water, so increasing their weight, and are used in foods such as frozen poultry and cured meats.

KEY POINTS

- Food additives prolong the shelf-life of foods and make them more appealing to eat.
- If you are concerned about the safety of additives, check food labels carefully.

Food allergies and intolerances

Food allergies and intolerances cause similar symptoms, but involve different mechanisms. Food allergies are caused by the immune system reacting abnormally to food. Most food could trigger an allergic response, but preparation, cooking and the action of digestive acid and enzymes destroy most of this potential.

When your body's defence system meets a potentially harmful substance, it responds with an immunological reaction. This releases histamine and other chemicals into your circulation, causing itching of the skin and changes in blood vessels. In serious cases, the changes in blood vessels can lead to a rapid fall in blood volume and a dramatic, and potentially fatal, reaction, known as anaphylactic shock, which can interfere with a person's ability to breathe. These chemicals also cause constriction of lung tissues and are associated with asthma.

Food intolerances do not involve an immunological reaction. Some of the mechanisms involved are not fully understood. Food intolerance reactions include:

COMMON ALLERGENS
Shellfish and strawberries are two of the most common foods responsible for true food allergies, which involve the immune system.

- **Non-allergic histamine release** Shellfish and strawberries cause this reaction in some people, who usually develop a rash.
- **Enzyme defects** People with a lactase deficiency, for example, are unable to digest the milk sugar lactose. The treatment consists of a diet low in milk and milk products.
- **Pharmacological reactions** These occur in response to food components, such as amines. Amines are found in foods that contain nitrogen (for example, amino acids in foods such as tea, coffee, cola drinks and chocolate). The effects may be triggered by small amounts of food and include migraine, tremor, sweating and palpitations, which can be alarming.
- **Irritant effects** Foods such as curry can irritate the gut. Monosodium glutamate can cause a condition known as Chinese restaurant syndrome, which results in chest pain, palpitations and weakness.

DIETARY TREATMENT

Anyone suspected of having a food allergy must be diagnosed and treated by a dietitian. Diagnosis is often based on eliminating possible allergens – substances that cause an allergic reaction – from the diet. An elimination diet is sometimes based on the very few foods that are unlikely to cause allergic reactions. This very limited diet is difficult to plan and stick to.

As each food is gradually reintroduced to the diet, a dietitian can assess which of them is responsible for any symptoms. This process needs careful monitoring. It is not safe to try excluding suspect foods from your diet by yourself. If it is necessary to use a very restrictive diet, there is a risk of nutritional deficiencies developing, unless it is carefully controlled. This is especially important in children, who need an adequate supply of the right nutrients in order to grow normally and maintain good health. The danger of anaphylaxis, or other severe reactions associated with the diagnosis of food allergy, means that the dietitian works closely with medical colleagues.

PREVENTING FOOD ALLERGIES

Some food allergies are inherited or may be related to a child becoming sensitised while in the womb or in the first months after birth.

ATOPIC ECZEMA

Atopic eczema affects children with a family history of allergies, including hay fever and asthma, and has been linked to food allergies. Some people have suggested that pregnant and breast-feeding women should change their diets to reduce or prevent the risk of their children developing allergies to foods. Mothers of children at risk of developing atopic eczema (the kind that runs in families, often together with asthma) should try to avoid highly allergenic foods such as milk and milk products, nuts, eggs and soya beans. It may also be worth delaying the introduction of any of these foods to the children until they are over eight months old. Breast milk appears to give some protection, but no one is sure whether cows' milk plays any role in triggering allergies.

Lactose Intolerance

People with lactase deficiency should avoid the products listed below. Several lactose-reduced milks and products are available commercially.

- Cows', goats' and sheep's milk.
- Milk products, such as cheese and skimmed milk.
- Milk derivatives often used in food manufacture, such as casein and hydrolysed whey. Remember to read the list of ingredients.
- Foods such as stock cubes and crisps, which often contain whey.
- Medicines that use milk products as fillers.

Despite an increase in breast-feeding in the UK, atopic eczema is more common than it used to be.

NUT ALLERGY

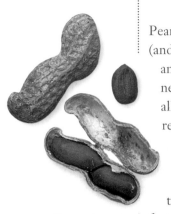

Peanuts are the most common cause of the serious (and sometimes fatal) allergic reaction known as anaphylaxis. Immediate medical attention is usually needed, although some people who are aware of their allergy carry medication to counteract their body's response. Not all peanut allergy sufferers have such a dramatic and rapid allergic reaction.

Recent studies have shown that peanut allergy is more common than previously realised and appears to be on the increase. This is probably related to the fact that women often eat larger quantities of peanuts and products containing peanut oil while pregnant or breast-feeding. Peanut and other nut allergies can be inherited, and any women with a family history of this type of allergy should avoid these foods during pregnancy and breast-feeding.

PEANUT ALLERGY
Peanuts can cause a severe, life-threatening allergy in some individuals.

HYPERACTIVITY

A link between hyperactive children and food additives was first suggested in the 1970s and has since gained popular support. Some scientists have found the behaviour of these children improved when some foods are eliminated from the diet. These include milk, eggs, wheat, nuts and colourings and preservatives such as tartrazine and benzoic acid. There is a link between food and hyperactivity in a minority of children, especially those with allergic conditions such as asthma and eczema. However, there is no conclusive evidence that any food is responsible for triggering the behaviour of most hyperactive children.

Case History: COELIAC DISEASE

Margaret was experiencing tiredness, weight loss, abdominal pain and diarrhoea, with bulky, foul-smelling stools that were difficult to flush away. Blood tests showed that she was anaemic, with iron and folate deficiencies. A tissue sample taken from her jejunum (small intestine) showed that her intestinal wall was flat with few of the characteristic projections called villi.

Margaret had a condition called coeliac disease. The wall of her jejunum was reacting to gluten, a constituent of wheat, as if it was toxic. Gluten makes wheat products such as cake and bread rise. The flattening of the villi meant that Margaret was unable to absorb nutrients properly, resulting in weight loss and deficiencies, causing anaemia and diarrhoea. The bulky, offensive stools were caused by a failure to absorb fat properly. They were difficult to flush away because of their high fat content.

Margaret's doctor prescribed iron and folate supplements to cure the anaemia and referred her to a dietitian specialising in gastrointestinal problems. She began a gluten-free diet, avoiding all products containing wheat, rye and barley. The dietitian told Margaret that not everyone agrees with the need to avoid oats, but suggested that she do so to begin with. Later, she could put them back on the menu to see whether her symptoms then recurred. A gluten-free diet is not easy to follow, because products such as flour are included in many food products as a thickening agent. Even small quantities of gluten may cause trouble to coeliac patients.

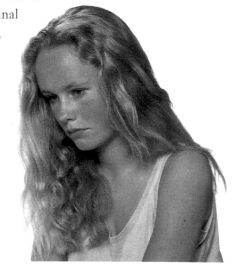

GLUTEN REACTION
Margaret's symptoms included extreme tiredness and abdominal pain. Tissue samples showed that her intestine was reacting adversely to gluten.

Margaret found it was essential to read food labels and obtained gluten-free food lists from the Coeliac Society. Her GP was able to prescribe gluten-free products.

Margaret's symptoms took several months to improve. She will have to remain on the diet for life to get permanent relief of her symptoms.

Case History: **LACTOSE INTOLERANCE**

Ken was admitted to a specialist nutrition unit because he was seriously obese. He was assessed to see whether he was suitable for a controversial treatment that involved wiring his jaw so that his mouth could open only very slightly. Ken had never particularly liked milk, but was resigned to the fact that, if he did have his jaws wired, it would become a major component of his diet. It was decided to go ahead with the treatment. Under medical supervision, Ken started a diet based on full-fat milk. Shortly afterwards, he developed nausea, bloating, abdominal pain and diarrhoea. It was discovered that Ken was intolerant to the milk sugar lactose. The dietitian devised another diet for Ken based on fermented milk products, such as yoghurt.

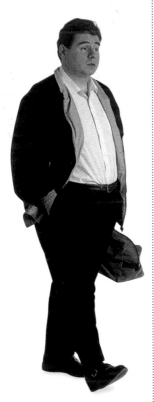

LACTOSE INTOLERANCE
A change in Ken's diet revealed a previously unrecognized intolerance to the milk sugar lactose.

KEY POINTS

- Food allergies involve immunological reactions; food intolerances involve many different non-immunological mechanisms, some of which are not fully understood.

- Never put your child on a restricted diet, even if you suspect an allergy, without getting expert advice first, no matter how mild the symptoms.

Supplements, diets and 'health foods'

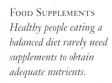

The growing interest in diet and health has stimulated an increase in the market for dietary supplements. The range of supplements available in health food shops, chemists and supermarkets is growing, with vitamins, minerals, fish liver oils and evening primrose oil being the most popular.

Dietary supplements fall between medicines and foods in terms of legal controls, and it is therefore difficult to regulate the way that they are promoted and sold. Some manufacturers make misleading claims about what their products can do and provide little, if any, information on possible side-effects and the hazards of overdosing. No medical claims can legally be made for these products unless they have been thoroughly tested and licensed.

FOOD SUPPLEMENTS
Healthy people eating a balanced diet rarely need supplements to obtain adequate nutrients.

NUTRIENT SUPPLEMENTS

The role of vitamins and minerals is well established (see 'Vitamins and minerals' on p.52). However, the use of large doses is controversial. Most people living in the UK should not need to take supplements to avoid becoming deficient in vitamins or minerals. A balanced diet will provide nutrients in sufficient quantities to satisfy your body's requirements. The only people who need supplements are those who suffer from medical conditions affecting their absorption or metabolism of certain nutrients.

The need to supplement the diet of pregnant women with folate and iron is one of the few exceptions. Folate supplementation before conception and in early pregnancy has been shown to reduce the incidence of neural tube defects such as spina bifida. The need to take iron in pregnancy is not totally accepted by doctors; some argue that the low blood concentrations of iron are due to a normal dilution by the increased blood volume that occurs in pregnancy. The amount of iron normally taken by pregnant women does not, however, appear to cause side-effects so, although it may not always do any good, it does no harm either.

Many other supplements make claims that have little or no scientific justification. Pyridoxine supplements are taken by many women to reduce symptoms associated with premenstrual syndrome, although there is no conclusive evidence to show that they work. Some research studies have shown that daily doses of 500 milligrams or more over several months may damage nerves in the feet and hands.

There is no evidence to support the theory that giving children vitamin supplements will make them more intelligent. All children need a balanced diet to function normally and to grow properly, and any dietary problems will obviously undermine their ability to do their school work well.

The Consumers Association has recently called for tighter controls on dietary supplements:

- Dietary supplements should be classified within food legislation and the Department of Health should be responsible for regulation.
- There should be specific labelling requirements and quality assurance regulations.
- Health claims should be supported by independent scientific research.
- Maximum doses should be specified.
- Rules for the notification of side-effects should be introduced, similar to the established procedure used for medicines.

HIGH-ENERGY SUPPLEMENTS

These products are aimed at exercise enthusiasts who want to eat more calories as they use up more energy. These people are often trying to increase their muscle mass and will require more protein. Calories are used mainly by lean tissue, of which muscle is a major component. As the muscle mass increases, more calories are needed to maintain the more muscular frame. However, these extra calories and protein can easily be supplied by eating more food. Elderly convalescents and their carers may also use these supplements. Although they may be of some benefit, their strong flavourings and rich nature make them unpalatable to people with poor appetites. It is usually better to offer convalescents frequent, small snacks and meals consisting of foods that they like and therefore will eat.

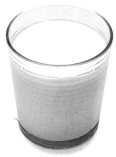

HIGH-ENERGY DRINKS
High-energy supplements are often made up with milk to increase their calorie content. They make a good supplement for the sports enthusiast.

'HEALTH FOODS'

This term is usually used to describe foods that are not readily available in supermarkets, but which are sold in specialist shops. The name implies that these foods are particularly healthy. This is misleading, as people who already eat a balanced diet are unlikely to derive any benefit from them. However, there are many useful products sold in health food shops. Wholemeal foods are a good example, although you can normally buy them just as easily in your local supermarket. Organic foods such as cereals, fruit and vegetables are becoming more widely available in both specialist shops and supermarkets, but they are invariably more expensive as a result of higher production costs. The use of natural farming methods has obvious advantages in reducing the reliance on pesticides and fertilisers. However, there is little scientific evidence to support the theory that organic foods are healthier than those produced by modern methods.

ALTERNATIVE DIETS

People are always looking to optimise the benefits from their diet. This has resulted in an increase in the number of people willing to pay for alternative diets, many of which are expensive with debatable, if any, benefits.

DETOXIFICATION DIETS

These are recommended by various health writers and therapists to cleanse the body, and often involve fasting, bathing and exfoliating (removal of dead skin by rubbing and brushing) to remove toxins. If your liver and kidneys are functioning properly, your body will clear any waste substances naturally. There is no scientific evidence to support the benefits of these diets. Always consult your medical practitioner before trying one of them.

ANTI-CANDIDA DIETS

It has been suggested that overgrowth of yeasts, particularly *Candida albicans*, can lead to a variety of debilitating symptoms. This overgrowth is supposedly triggered by diets rich in yeasts and sugar (which is used as food by yeasts), oral contraceptives and the use of broad-spectrum antibiotics. This is alleged to result in toxin production, which weakens the immune system, making susceptible people prone to a wide range of illnesses. The diet used to treat this condition involves avoiding bread, vinegar, alcohol, pickles, cheese, yeast extracts and all products containing sucrose. There is no medically controlled evidence to justify the use of these diets.

Food-combining (Hay) Diet

Supporters of these diets claim that the body cannot digest acid and alkaline foods together. They also claim that mixing protein and carbohydrate foods results in many health problems, such as headaches, allergies and obesity. In reality, the digestive system is fully capable of digesting a meal containing a mixture of foods using varying acid and alkaline conditions.

Slimming Diets

There are many diets that are supposed to make it easy for people to lose weight. Many totally eliminate one food group from the diet. It is suggested that these diets 'burn fat' or 'speed up the metabolism'. Some slimming diets are based on single foods, such as grapefruit. Such claims have no scientific basis and, if you succeed in losing weight, it is because of their restrictive nature. These diets will not help you change to a healthy eating pattern in the long term. They can also cause nutritional deficiencies.

Very-low-calorie diets (VLCD) were very popular in the 1980s and provided less than 400 kcal per day. Medical evidence linked these diets to cardiac problems.

A Government committee recommended that these diets should not be used for longer than 3–4 weeks and then only by obese people under medical supervision. The energy content and presentation of these diets were then changed to provide 600–800 kcal per day, incorporating snack bars and prepared meals. Their popularity has greatly declined.

Low-carbohydrate diets were most popular in the 1960s. Reducing your intake of carbohydrate leads to the mobilisation of fat stores, releasing chemicals called ketones. Ketones are made from the breakdown of fat and can be used by the body, but not the brain, as an energy source for a limited period. These diets were successful in restricting energy intake, as many people would find it difficult to eat large amounts of fat or protein without carbohydrate. The lack of carbohydrate results in the rapid use of glycogen energy stores. This also causes the loss of water, which accounts for the initial rapid weight loss. When carbohydrate is reintroduced, weight gain occurs.

The best approach to losing weight is to adopt a healthy diet. This will make sure your weight remains as it should be in the long term, as well as providing all the nutrients you need for good health (see 'Healthy eating' on p.63).

Case History: **LOSS OF APPETITE**

At 74, Sophie was becoming frail. She had recently had major surgery and had gone to stay with her daughter to convalesce. Her daughter Hilary and her family were health conscious and had a varied, balanced, high-fibre, low-fat diet. Hilary used a lot of wholemeal products, especially pasta and granary breads. Hilary believed that this diet would speed up her mother's recovery.

Unfortunately, Sophie's appetite was poor and she was becoming increasingly uninterested in food. She did not like pasta, preferring more 'traditional' meals. The district nurse advised Hilary to talk to the dietitian at the local health centre. She recommended giving Sophie meals that she would eat and enjoy rather than providing 'healthy' foods. The dietitian also advised Hilary to:

- Remember that high-energy supplements can be overwhelming and very filling. Milky drinks are often a more acceptable alternative.
- Give plenty of fluids, but not immediately before a meal as they may reduce the appetite.
- Ask Sophie's doctor whether vitamin supplements would be helpful; some prescribed drugs can interact with nutrients in the diet or affect absorption.
- Take care when reducing fat in her diet as this may affect her vitamin D and calcium levels.

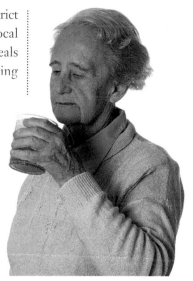

Hilary began providing smaller meals of simple dishes that Sophie preferred to pasta and granary bread. Sophie found that she liked a hot chocolate Complan drink supplement before bed. Once Sophie's appetite had returned, Hilary was able to increase the portions so that her mother gradually gained weight.

MILKY DRINK
A high energy milk drink, together with traditional home cooking, helped to build up Sophie after she underwent major surgery.

KEY POINTS

- The use of food supplements is often unnecessary.
- Normal foods can be modified to provide any additional requirements.
- Lack of appetite is an important factor when trying to persuade someone to eat more.
- Most healthy people are unlikely to experience any specific nutrient deficiency.

Useful addresses

British Allergy Foundation
30 Bellgrove Road
Welling
Kent DA16 3PY
Tel: (020) 8303 8525
Helpline: (020) 8303 8583
Provides information on
allergies.

British Diabetic Association
10 Queen Anne Street
London W1M 0BD
Tel: (020) 7323 1531
Helpline: (020) 7636 6112
Provides information and
support for people with
diabetes and their families.

British Heart Foundation
14 Fitzhardinge Street
London W1H 4DH
Tel: (020) 7935 0185
Provides information and
support for people with heart
conditions and their families.

**The British Nutrition
Foundation**
High Holborn House
52–54 High Holborn
London WC1V 6RQ
Tel: (020) 7404 6504
A science charity providing free
factsheets and publications lists.

The Coeliac Society
PO Box 220
High Wycombe
Bucks HP11 2HY
Tel: (01494) 437 278
Provides information and
support for people with
coeliac disease.

**Hyperactive Children's
Support Group**
17 Whyke Lane
Chichester
West Sussex PO19 2LD
Provides information and
support for parents with a
hyperactive child.

National Asthma Campaign
Providence House
Providence Place
London N1 0NT
Tel: (01345) 010203 (Weekdays
13:00–21:00)
Provides information and
support for people with asthma.

Vegan Society
Donald Wilson House
7 Battle Road
St. Leonards-on-Sea
East Sussex TN37 7AA
Tel: (01424) 427 393
Send large SAE for information.

Vegetarian Society
Parkdale
Dunham Road
Altrincham
Cheshire WA14 4QG
Tel: (0161) 928 0793
Provides a starter pack for
vegetarians; send an A5 SAE
for a list of local groups.

Government Publications
Department of Health
PO Box 410
Wetherby LS23 7LN

Health Education Authority
Customer Services
Marston Book Services Ltd
PO Box 269
Abingdon
Oxon OX14 4YN
Tel: (01235) 465565

**Ministry of Agriculture,
Food and Fisheries (MAFF)**
Tel: (0645) 556000
Publications available from
FOOD SENSE:
London SE99 2TT

Glossary

amino acid: an organic acid that combines with other amino acids to form proteins

atom: the smallest unit of a substance; atoms combine to make molecules

BMI: body mass index (weight in kg/[height in m]^2)

BMR: basal metabolic rate; the rate at which the body uses energy at complete rest

enzyme: proteins that regulate biological reactions and are essential for digestion; specific enzymes are responsible for the breakdown of certain foods; for example, lipases break down fats into fatty acids

CHD: coronary heart disease

EAR: estimated average requirement of a group of people for energy, protein or a vitamin or mineral

fatty acid: basic units that combine to form fats (lipids)

fibre: see NSP

kcal: kilocalorie; a unit used to measure the energy value of food

kJ: kilojoule or 1,000 joules; a unit used to measure the energy value of food (1 kcal = 4.18 kJ)

lipids: a collective word for fats and oils

MJ: megajoule or 1 million joules

molecules: large compounds formed from small units

NSPs: non-starch polysaccharides; commonly referred to as fibre

peristalsis: the movement of food along the intestine caused by the wave-like contraction of muscles in the intestinal wall

RDA: recommended daily amounts of food energy and nutrients for groups of people

RNI: reference nutrient intake

saccharide: the basic unit of carbohydrates; they exist singularly as monosaccharides or combine to form larger molecules such as disaccharides, starches and polysaccharides

vegetarian: a diet, or someone eating that diet, that does not include meat; it may include eggs, milk and sometimes fish

vegan: a diet that contains absolutely no animal products, or someone eating that diet

Index

Acknowledgements

PUBLISHER'S ACKNOWLEDGEMENTS
Dorling Kindersley would like to thank the following for their help
and participation in this project:

DTP Jason Little;
Consultancy Dr. Sue Davidson; **Indexing** Indexing Specialists, Hove
Administration Christopher Gordon.

Photography Paul Mattock; Ian Parsons. **Illustrations** (p.20) © Richard Tibbits.
Picture Research Andy Samson; **Picture Librarian** Charlotte Oster.

PICTURE CREDITS
The publisher would like to thank the following for their kind
permission to reproduce their photographs. Every effort has been made
to trace the copyright holders. Dorling Kindersley apologises for any
unintentional omissions and would be pleased, in any such cases,
to add an acknowledgement in future editions.

Family Life Picture Library p.32 (Angela Hampton); **Format Photographers** p.61
(Paula Solloway): **Robert Harding Picture Library** p.52 (David A. wagner); **Holt Studios
International** p.25 (Nigel Cattlin); **Science Photo Library** p.9 (Dr Klaus Shiller).